RECENT ADVANCES IN PEDIATRIC CLINICAL PATHOLOGY

C. Charlton Mabry, M.D., M.S. (Ped.), F.A.A.P.

> *Associate Professor of Pediatrics and Assistant Pathologist, University of Kentucky, Lexington, Kentucky*

Irene E. Roeckel, M.D., F.C.A.P., F.A.S.C.P.

> *Associate Professor of Pathology and Assistant Pathologist, University of Kentucky, Lexington, Kentucky*

Robert E. Gevedon, B.S., M.T. (ASCP), A.A.C.C.

> *Assistant Chief Medical Technologist (Chemistry), University Hospital, Lexington, Kentucky*

John A. Koepke, M.D., M.S. (Path.), F.C.A.P., F.A.S.C.P.

> *Associate Professor of Pathology and Associate Pathologist, University of Kentucky, Lexington, Kentucky*

 GRUNE & STRATTON   **NEW YORK AND LONDON**

Portions of this book were aided by U. S. Public Health Service Research Grant HD-00040 from the National Institute of Child Health and Human Development.

Contents

Preface

THE ORIGINAL VERSION of this manual was prepared to provide instruction material for a postgraduate course held at the University of Kentucky in the Spring of 1967. Further revision and updating of the manual was made to prepare it for use in a national workshop sponsored by the American Society of Clinical Pathologists in the Fall of 1967. The clinical chemistry determinations considered are those most frequently requested; they constitute the "core" of chemical tests expected of a University Hospital central laboratory. Automated micro methods are used for all patients, pediatric and adult, in our laboratory. The methods described are in current day to day use. An alternate manual micro method follows when it is used on occasion in our laboratory. For the special chemistry procedures presented, rapidity and ease of performance are emphasized.

The format is designed to keep the manual simple and of handbook size. Tests that frequently are requested together, that are related to similar disorders, or that involve similar metabolites are grouped into chapters. If the user has had some experience with laboratory procedures, the protocols provided are sufficient. Each chapter begins with a discussion of clinical usefulness, collection precautions, and interpretation of values of the tests described.

The impetus for preparing this manual was the introduction of micro adaptations of the most-used AutoAnalyzer methods and the transfer of a number of special chemistry tests from our research laboratories to the central clinical laboratory. These new or special methods, in large part, have been developed by the authors or others on our staff. Importantly, by adhering to the central laboratory concept, many tests are now available to all patients. In addition, our laboratory liaison service is described. It has insured complete and accurate collection of all specimens and has provided results which are posted on individual patient charts within several hours.

We are indebted to the entire staff of the Central Clinical Laboratory of the University Hospital. Without their aid and tolerance, this manual could not have been developed. Those who made unique and special contributions are Elizabeth Austin, Robert Blackburn, Julianne Harris, Reedes Hurt, Betty Mulberry, Peggy Warth and Denver Robertson. Editorially, we are indebted to Barbara Mabry, Ann Perkins and Donna Taylor. Finally, the satisfaction of working together has been our greatest personal reward.

C. Charlton Mabry, M.D.

Irene E. Roeckel, M.D.

Robert E. Gevedon, B.S., M.T. (ASCP)

John A. Koepke, M.D.

Lexington, Kentucky

Foreword
For the Benefit of Children

WHEN I BEGAN negotiations to join the University of Kentucky five years ago, I was assured that the hospital's pediatric service, though small, had the benefit of micro-chemical methods. At the demand of the pediatricians, a number of manual micro-sample procedures had just been established in the Central Clinical Laboratory. By the time I had moved to Lexington, three months later, this adaptation of the laboratory to children had vanished. The University of Kentucky Hospital, it turned out, at the time was no different from many other hospitals; it had proved unsound in a general hospital to provide special methods for children. In a laboratory geared to adults, automated methods were a financial necessity.

It mattered not that the amount of blood requested by the laboratory to perform a glucose tolerance test for a premature was one-tenth of his total blood volume. Nor did it matter that venipunctures of femoral veins subjected newborns to the risk of a low but intolerable incidence of osteomyelitis, which was rarely mentioned. Nor did it matter that physicians tended to settle for less than ideal investigation of sick babies because it was too time consuming and inconvenient for them to personally draw venous blood samples which laboratory girls could not be expected to draw. In that day and age it was simply not practical for the general hospital laboratory to cater to a small number of children.

The University of Kentucky was fortunate to have the authors of this book on its staff. Dedicated to the idea that children are more important than anybody, and that somehow we ought to be nice to them and protect them from painful and frightening experiences when they are sick, these workers came up with the logical solution—*use methods designed for children for everybody!* This solution seems so simple that many visitors to our institution think that we must have settled for lesser accuracy. They have to be shown that this is not so.

The authors are well qualified to have accomplished this simple solution. Dr. Mabry, for instance, is a pediatrician by training, a chemist-pediatrician whose investigative work lies in the area of metabolic diseases, inborn errors of metabolism, and genetics. Many of the analytic methods in his type of research laboratory require the smallest of samples. As a clinician dealing with remote mountain families with children having PKU, he needed a way for mothers to draw blood samples and mail them to the University to monitor the dietary management of their children. So he devised a method to suit his requirements. He was one of the early American workers to exploit the potentialities of high voltage electrophoresis. Brought up in the research laboratory, he is devoted to accuracy rather than expediency.

As the Director of the Children's Medical Service and as an attending physician on the childrens' wards of the University of Kentucky Medical Center, I see evidence daily that the availability of these methods and the collection of capillary blood samples by friendly girls who get along well with children lead to better medical care for children. It is my sincere hope that these methods will spread widely and that as a result better medical care can be brought to children everywhere.

> Warren E. Wheeler, M.D.
> Professor and Chairman
> Department of Pediatrics
> University of Kentucky
> Director of Pediatric Service
> University of Kentucky Hospital

As Dr. Wheeler mentioned in his portion of the foreword, due to restrictions in space, personnel and funds, it is nearly impractical for a clinical laboratory in an active general hospital to provide different methods of performing clinical laboratory examinations for children and adults. The obvious solution has been found, namely: adapting all the methods to small samples suitable to children. This the authors have accomplished almost entirely through their own efforts, but with some early assistance from members of the Technicon Corporation. Basically, what they have done is modify, occasionally extensively, methods used in the routine chemistry laboratory so that no single determination or group of determinations requires more than one-tenth of a milliliter of serum. The accuracy and precision of these methods has been carefully explored over the years and there is reason to believe they are actually superior to the standard methods.

The members of the Department of Pathology who were involved in this development and are co-authors of the text are, by their background and training well equiped to perform this function. Dr. Roeckel received her medical education in Heidelberg, Germany, and immigrated to this country shortly after World War II, following internship and various research posts at Heidelberg University. She took further training in the United States at Delafield Hospital, Columbia University, in New York City, and at the Emergency Hospital in Washington, D. C. She served as an assistant Professor of Pathology at Georgetown University and joined the University of Kentucky faculty in 1964, where she is now an associate professor. Ever since joining us, she has been professionally responsible for the clinical chemistry laboratory.

Dr. Koepke received his medical education at the University of Wisconsin, his intern and residency training in Milwaukee, associated with Marquette University. He joined the faculty at Kentucky in 1961 as an assistant professor and became an associate professor in January 1965. He has been in charge of the hematology and special chemistry sections of the clinical laboratory ever since he arrived and has also proved to be an active investigator.

Mr. Gevedon is a medical technologist and at the time these procedures were developed was assistant chief medical technologist for chemistry, in charge of the automated area.

Through the efforts of these individuals and all other personnel in the laboratory, we have been able to provide more than satisfactory service for the children and at the same time improve our services to adults. This illustrates the advances possible in patient care when there exists close collaboration and interchange of information between the laboratory and clinical services.

W. B. Stewart, M. D.
Professor and Chairman
Department of Pathology
University of Kentucky
Director of Laboratory Services
University of Kentucky Hospital

Introduction

AUTOMATIC CHEMICAL ANALYSIS AND MICROCHEMISTRIES

THE USE OF only small amounts of blood for clinical chemistry tests is a continuing goal in patient care. Moreover, there is a conspicuous advantage in using capillary blood from infants, children, and even some adults. Manual micro- and ultramicrochemistries, introduced a decade ago for infants and children, have not stood the test of time in the work-a-day clinical laboratory; they are cumbersome, time consuming and less accurate than macro and semi-micro methods. With the offering of a larger variety of tests and their greatly increased use, there is an even greater need to reduce the amount of blood required for laboratory tests on all patients. To meet this pressing need for small sample size and rapid test performance on large numbers of samples, we have capitalized on a newly emerging technology—continuous-flow chemistry or in-stream analysis.

This ingenious system of continuous-flow analysis, employing conventional and classical methods for the determination of various constituents in blood, was described by L. T. Skeggs a decade ago. Now available commercially as the Technicon AutoAnalyzer, the apparatus is capable of performing many different techniques in chemical analysis. In-stream analysis utilizes a constant rate of liquid flow within glass and plastic tubing, with all chemical reactions taking place in these flowing streams. One analysis follows the next down the stream; reagents are added from side streams as needed. Samples are dialyzed, heated, and mixed according to the requirements of the method. The sensing devices used in our adapted methods are colorimeters, fluorometers, and a flame photometer. All of the reactions are completely automatic; the end results are registered by strip-chart recorders. Most of the AutoAnalyzer methods employ 0.3 to 2.0 ml of sample; we have adapted or introduced new methods for direct use of 0.1 ml or less plasma or serum for groups of the most frequently used clinical biochemical analyses.

The development of this system of automatic analysis has several signficant implications for the medical profession. First, by relieving the tedium of routine manual determinations, it is possible to decrease considerably the amount of technician time per analysis. In our laboratory it has already been shown that there will not be a decrease in the required number of technicians, but rather a dramatic increase in number of tests ordered and in the output of analytical data. Second, by decreasing the time interval between sampling and result, the utility of the analytical data is greatly increased. Third, tests that are so cumbersome as not to warrant routine application if handled manually can frequently be adapted and performed with ease. Fourth, the inherent precision and visual record of work performed enhances the confidence

1

in the data. Fifth, these adaptations to micro samples have provided, for the first time, reliable microchemistry data from a central clinical laboratory where technologists rotate work assignments. Moreover, since most infants and children are hospitalized in general hospitals, the pediatric needs are best served where the entire hospital utilizes microchemistries.

Naturally, the problems involved in micro-automation of a clinical chemistry laboratory touch all facets of patient care. Some educators and physicians are disturbed because this easy availability of laboratory data is altering the traditional approach in making diagnoses and managing patients. The ultimate utility of this or any other system of automation is directly related to the ingenuity and thoughtfulness of both the chemist and the physician at the ground level of their everyday activities. We would view the methods and services outlined in this manual as medical advances, and the new diagnostic approaches and patterns of patient care that evolve are improvements and best for most patients.

REFERENCE
1. Skeggs, Jr., L. T.: An automatic method for colorimetric analysis. Am. J. Clin. Path. 28: 311–322, 1957.

COLLECTION AND PROCESSING OF SPECIMENS

In the use and interpretation of laboratory data for the diagnosis and management of disease many factors come into play. When errors arise, one thinks immediately that the analysis itself or the computation of the results is incorrect. Just as important in this respect, however, are errors which arise from improper collection and preservation of specimens for analysis. In our experience, this area has been responsible for the largest number of errors. Moreover, it is in the area of collection of specimens and reporting of results in which the clinical pathologist and laboratory technologist frequently find themselves in conflict with the patient's clinician. Collection of specimens and reporting of results requires unusual interdisciplinary cooperation when the numbers of specimens on individual patients are large. In the past, a patient either in the clinic or in the hospital had only a few laboratory determinations. In a university hospital the average number of clinical chemistry tests per patient admission is about 15, with every indication that both the number of tests on individual patients and the number of patients seeking service are rapidly increasing. For these reasons, the clinical laboratory must assume a more complete responsibility for laboratory determinations from the time that they are ordered to the time that they are posted in the individual patient's chart, thus making them available for the clinician's easy and timely use. The following section includes a description both of our method of controlling the collection and the final reporting of results in our hospital and of the techniques of collection and preservation of specimens.

A. Laboratory Liaison Service

This part of our laboratory service consolidates many services that traditionally have been performed by nurses and physicians. A laboratory order

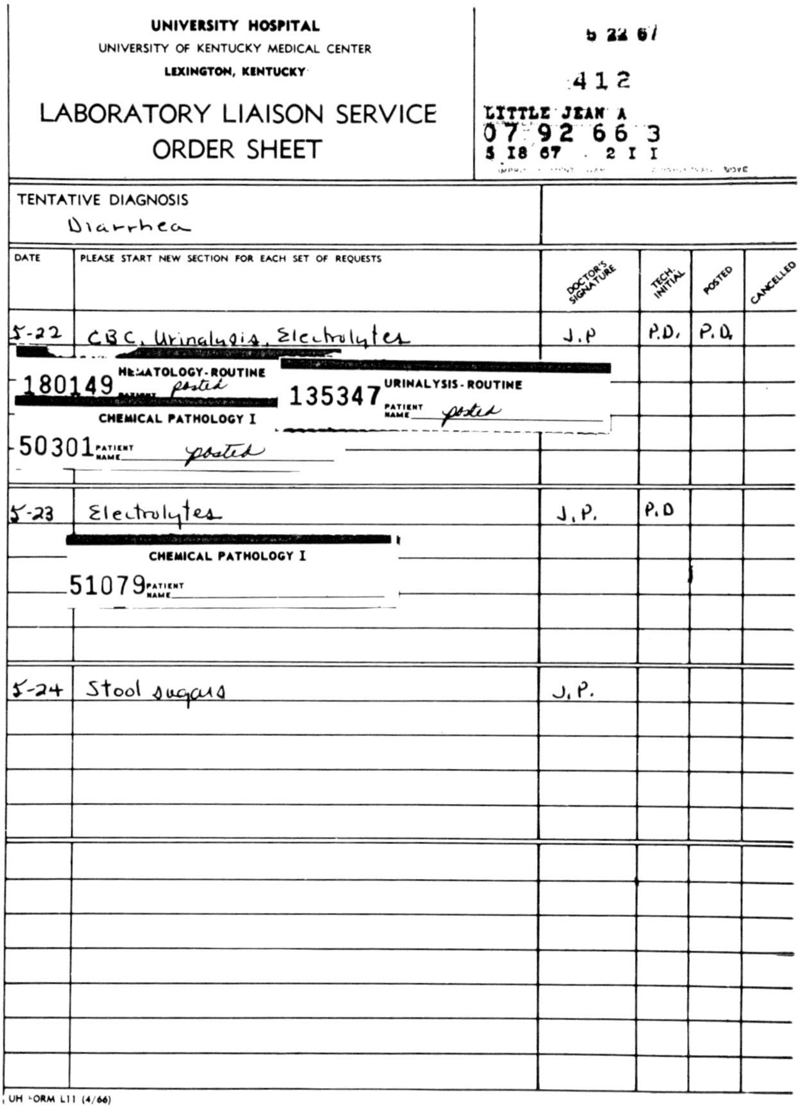

UNIVERSITY HOSPITAL
UNIVERSITY OF KENTUCKY MEDICAL CENTER
LEXINGTON, KENTUCKY

LABORATORY LIAISON SERVICE
ORDER SHEET

b 22 67

412

LITTLE JEAN A
07 92 66 3
5 18 67 · 2 I I

TENTATIVE DIAGNOSIS					
Diarrhea					

DATE	PLEASE START NEW SECTION FOR EACH SET OF REQUESTS	DOCTOR'S SIGNATURE	TECH INITIAL	POSTED	CANCELLED
5-22	CBC, Urinalysis, Electrolytes	J.P	P.D.	P.D.	
	HEMATOLOGY-ROUTINE *posted* 135347 URINALYSIS-ROUTINE *posted*				
180149	CHEMICAL PATHOLOGY I				
50301	PATIENT NAME *posted*				
5-23	Electrolytes	J.P.	P.D		
	CHEMICAL PATHOLOGY I				
51079	PATIENT NAME				
5-24	Stool sugars	J.P.			

UH FORM L11 (4/66)

Fig. Intro-1. Physician laboratory order sheet; monitored and maintained by Laboratory Liaison Technician.

book is maintained at each hospital nursing station, with separate physician order sheets inserted for each patient. The laboratory liaison technician is responsible for (1) acknowledging each request, (2) completing each test requisition form, (3) obtaining and submitting the specimen for analysis, and (4) entering the results in the individual patient charts. The laboratory liaison technician's performance is enhanced by use of a cart efficiently equipped with the necessary clerical and technical supplies.

In many hospitals the laboratory technical staff has always been responsible for collecting blood specimens and returning all laboratory results to the nurs-

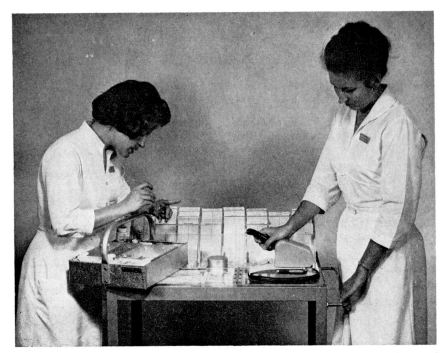

Fig. Intro-2. Liaison Technicians preparing laboratory requisitions and samples on cart.

ing stations at the end of the day. With an ever-increasing number of laboratory requests on individual patients, this traditional administrative scheme is unsuitable. The Laboratory Liaison Service we use supercedes former collection and reporting patterns in that (1) the laboratory assumes near total responsibility and control for all specimen collections; (2) personnel with practical nurse or limited technical skills are used, thus conserving laboratory and nursing professions; and (3) liaison personnel provide prompt posting of results in individual patient charts, resulting in a half-day collection to reporting cycle for most tests.

It has been estimated that as many as ten per cent of laboratory tests are either not timed, collected, or reported properly for use in patient care. Our system reduces this probability to a minimum and promotes more rapid patient "work-ups" and care decisions. For infants there is a special benefit in having only a few individuals responsible for specimen collections. Heel and finger puncture techniques to obtain blood are not difficult to learn, but they are skills that must be maintained by constant use. Also, this procedure is best done by individuals who are not rushed by other primary responsibilities.

B. Techniques of Specimen Collection and Preservation

1. Blood: Blood obtained by venipuncture or by capillary collection is suitable for the analysis of most blood constituents. Ideally, blood should be collected while the patient is in the fasting state, usually before breakfast. An-

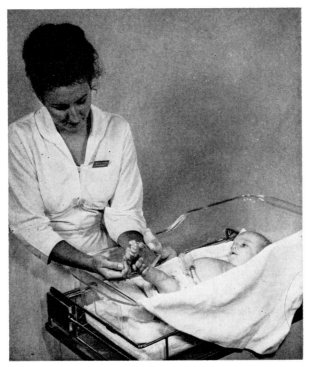

Fig. Intro-3. Liaison technician collecting capillary blood from an infant.

nino and Relman studied the effect of eating on some of the frequently ordered chemical constituents of blood; they concluded that in apparently normal persons probably none of the constituents, except glucose and inorganic phosphorus, will be affected 45 minutes to two hours after an average breakfast. Usually the practical problem is that in some adults their serum becomes lipemic following eating, and this may interfere with the analyses of many substances.

Ordinarily, for venipuncture a tourniquet is applied to the forearm and an antecubital vein becomes distended and visible. At the site of the venipuncture, 70 per cent alcohol is applied by sponge for cleansing and sterilization and allowed to evaporate. This ritual, however, does not completely disinfect the skin surface; it does have a psychologic effect and does cleanse skin which is particularly dirty. Blood collections from infants are obtained as capillary collections. The reason for obtaining capillary blood from infants and young children is that it is much less of a traumatic and hazardous experience than a femoral vein puncture or jugular vein "tap," and has the additional advantage that it can be repeated frequently. Sites in order of suitability are heel, big toe, fingertip and earlobe. The blood must flow freely, so a carefully chosen instrument must be used to rupture cleanly a great number of capillaries with a minimum of tissue trauma. It should be apparent that a certain depth must be obtained in an area of maximum capillarity so that, if this is achieved, the amount of blood flowing from the wound will only depend on the length of

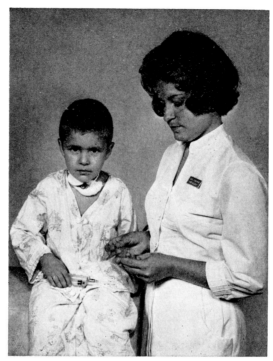

Fig. Intro-4. Liaison technician collecting capillary blood from a child. Compare the capillary collection tube being used with the conventional size collection syringes being held by child.

the wound and the speed of blood flow through the capillaries. If the punctured area has been previously arterialized by heating with a warm wash cloth, blood flow is enhanced. Cleansing agents that evaporate quickly (e.g., ether) excessively cool the skin and diminish arterialization.

A suggested procedure follows: Clean the area with 70 per cent alcohol and allow to dry. The use of 70 per cent alcohol will cause blood to spread and if any alcohol should come into contact with the blood, hemolysis will occur if the alcohol is not allowed to dry. The heel, toe or finger that is to be punctured is first warmed, cleansed with 70 per cent alcohol as needed; then a vertical push-puncture is then made with a #11 Bard Parker blade. To avoid hemolysis and contamination of the tissue fluid, it is essential to obtain a free flow of blood. This should require little or no "milking"; squeezing must not be resorted to at any time. The free-flowing blood is allowed to fill a Caraway micro-blood collecting tube by capillary action and gravity.

The collecting tube is heparinized prior to use with ammonium heparinate (sodium free); after use, the tapered end is occluded with vinyl plastic putty; the tube then is centrifuged at approximately 5000 × gravity for one minute*

---

*International Micro-Hematocrit, Centrifuge Model MB with 16-place head. Sample slots are milled down to base. Embroidery hoop used as gasket, because tapered ends of Caraway tubes cut standard rubber gasket.

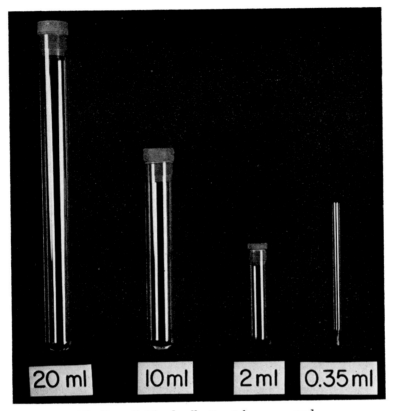

Fig. Intro-5. Blood collection tubes compared.

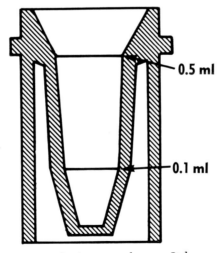

Fig. Intro-6. Cutaway view of micro sample cup. It has a conical bottom, ringed base for stability, collar on top for handling, and calibrations in 0.1 ml. increments. The small diameter promotes nearly complete utilization of sample with minimal evaporation loss.

and the supernatant plasma is transferred by a disposable long glass Pasteur pipette into a micro sample cup.° The maximum specimen volume of the sealed micro collecting tube† is 350 µL and should yield about 150 µL of plasma; care should be taken to fill each sample cup with at least 150µL of plasma. This new 500 µL capacity sample cup has a narrow internal diameter and conical bottom which provides a low surface-to-volume ratio. When venous blood is obtained, larger amounts of the sample may be placed in the specimen cup without altering the amount aspirated by the sample probe; the rapid entry and exit of the sampling needle precludes variable sampling times. The Sampler I module, with a slowly moving probe, aspirates slightly more or less of the sample in proportion to the height of the sample in the cup; hence, it is not suitable for these methods.

Serum is preferable to whole blood or to plasma for most biochemical analyses because (1) it is not subjected to variations in cell volume, (2) it is not contaminated with products of hemolysis, and (3) it is spared the effects of anticoagulants that may alter tests. However, the data obtained when certain anticoagulants are used is acceptable in most instances. The special care for certain determinations will be discussed under the individual methods. Ordinarily, serum or plasma should be separated from the cells as soon as practically feasible and the specimens stored frozen ($-10°$ C) unless noted otherwise.

2. Urine: In the collection of urine for chemistry tests, the most important problem revolves around the timing of a 24-hour urine collection and the preservation of the urine during and after the collection period. Even though a urine collection is timed, special care has to be used to make sure that the bladder was emptied prior to timing the urine collection. For the adult the 24-hour urine sample should be between 1,000 and 2,000 ml. in volume. Adult urine volumes of less than 500 or more than 3,000 ml. should be questioned in respect to their accuracy. Although these volumes are possible in certain clinical conditions, they are infrequent. Urine from infants is much smaller in volume and usually can be collected in small disposable plastic bags. Frequent changing of these plastic bags and pooling the voided urine is necessary in obtaining a prolonged urine collection.

Random urine collections may yield valid chemical data if creatinine levels are also measured. The constituent in question may be compared to the level of creatinine excretion since its excretion is constant in individual patients. Thus, creatinine excretion is a relatively constant reference.

By the careful use of cleansing methods with antiseptics, material approximating a "clean catch" specimen can be obtained for bacteriologic evaluation.

3. Spinal Fluid: Cerebral spinal fluid is essentially a dialysate or ultrafiltrate of blood. In part it also is a product of the secretory activity of the choroid plexus and may be preserved by the same techniques as for blood plasma or

---

°Distributed by Technicon Instruments Corporation, Ardsley, New York, Part No. 127093.

†No. A-2934, Clay-Adams, Inc., New York, New York 10010 (Length 75 mm, i.d. 2 mm, o.d. 4 mm).

serum. Often physicians fail to realize the necessity of relating normal values for cerebral spinal fluid constituents to the level of the spinal cord from which the fluid was withdrawn. Ventricular fluid contains a greater concentration of glucose than does lumbar fluid; conversely, ventricular fluid contains much less protein than does lumbar fluid. Also, the range of cerebral spinal fluid protein is greater in the newly born infant than in the older infant or child.

Spinal fluids taken as part of the diagnostic study of an individual who has had a convulsion should be compared with the serum sugar taken at the same time. Diagnostic lumbar punctures on chronically ill patients are frequently performed in the evening when the patient may continue his customary recumbent position and not be subject to post-lumbar tap headaches. A cell count and culture should be performed immediately, but glucose and protein determinations may wait until morning. The specimen should be frozen until shortly before the analysis.

REFERENCES

1. Annino, J. S., and Relman, A. S.: Effect of eating on some of the clinically important chemical constituents of the blood. Amer. J. Clin. Path. 31: 155–159, 1959.

2. Asnes, R. S., and Arendar, G. M.: Septic arthritis of the hip; a complication of femoral venipuncture. Pediatrics 38: 837–841, 1966.

3. DeChanar, C.: Cerebrospinal fluid, its physiology and diagnostic evaluation. Texas Rep. Bio. Med. 17: 453–466, 1959.

4. Hughes, Jr., W. T.: Collection of blood specimens. In *Pediatric Procedures.* Philadelphia: W. B. Saunders, 1964.

5. Kaplan, S. A., Yuceoglu, A. M., and Strauss, J.: Chemical microanalysis: analysis of capillary and venous blood. Pediatrics 24: 270–274, 1959.

6. McKay, Jr., R. J.: Risks of obtaining samples of venous blood in infants. Pediatrics 38: 906–908, 1966.

APPARATUS

The equipment, supplies and materials used in performing the procedures described in this manual, except for the continuous-flow analysis modules and the high-voltage electrophoresis equipment, are standard items in most clinical laboratories. An investment in so-called ultra-micro equipment and accessories is not required. Moreover, the use of continuous-flow analysis procedures requires a relatively small stock of pipettes of all sizes; a major saving in expendable glassware.

A. *Continuous-flow analysis equipment* is marketed as the AutoAnalyzer by Technicon Instrument Corp., Ardsley, N.Y. They supply detailed operational and maintenance instructions for the individual modules.

A brief description of the modules follows:

1. Sampler II: A circular sample plate with forty holes in the periphery is fitted to an indexing motor drive shaft. Individual samples are pipetted or poured into disposable plastic cups and the cups mounted in the holes of the plate. Analysis speed (20, 30, 40, 50, 60, 70, 120 per hour) is determined by interchangeable "cams." Sampling is accomplished by automatic rotation of a sample cup into position, dipping into a water wash, and rotation of the sample plate to the next position. The sample-to-wash time is usually a 2:1 ratio, but

this can be altered by changing the cam or by inserting water sample cups between samples. The usual procedure includes having standard solutions in five to ten cups of forty available cup positions. A cover is applied to the sample plate to prevent evaporation.

2. Proportioning pump: The pump is a peristaltic action type. A constant speed-motor chain drives a series of rollers sequentially across a springloaded plate. Compressed between the rollers and plate are, in parallel, as many as fifteen plastic tubes, the point of compression moving lengthwise along the tubes as the roller moves. When each roller lifts off the plate on completion of its compression stroke, the succeeding roller has compressed the tubes at a point further back, and the entrapped volume between the rollers is forced into the flow system. At constant pumping rate, the internal diameter of the tubes determines the volume flow of fluid through the tubes. The single pump therefore creates a continuous flow stream of reagent solutions on which is superimposed the intermittent sample flow. The volume of any reagent and the time of addition are determined, then, by the diameter of the tube used to pump that reagent and the position downstream at which the reagent is injected into the main stream. The volume of sample is determined by the diameter of tubing in the pump and by the sample rate. Air is employed in the main streams to compartmentalize liquid segments, which in turn helps reduce contamination between samples, presumably by a more discrete transport of the various fluids.

3. Dialyzer: The dialyzer consists of a cellophane sheet compressed between two plastic plates. The plastic plates have grooved channels through which fluid is pumped on either side of the membrane. The two fluids in the channels then both come in contact with opposite sides of the cellophane membrane, allowing dialysis to occur. The upper solution is generally the sample stream and the lower is either water or a reagent to act as recipient or acceptor of all materials dialyzed. In this continuous flow dialyzer, protein and cellular debris are separated from substances which are diffusable. Although the dialysis rate may be affected by many physical and chemical factors, sufficient control of these factors has been achieved in this flow stream dialyzer to maintain constant proportionality between the concentration of test substance in the sample stream and in the recipient stream. Fluctuations due to ambient temperature changes are kept to a minimum by immersing the dialyzer in a constant temperature bath.

4. Heating bath: In addition to the constant temperature bath necessary for maintenance of dialysis rate, other incubation or heating baths are available, though not necessary for all tests. Single coil and double coil baths have 480 to 920 inches of glass tubing respectively within the thermostatically controlled bath. For those tests requiring relatively high reaction temperatures, 95° C has been generally chosen to keep expansion of the air bubbles to a minimum and vaporization of water down to a point where surging of the solution leaving the bath does not destroy the segmentation phenomen established through the remainder of the system. For enzyme activity analysis, the bath

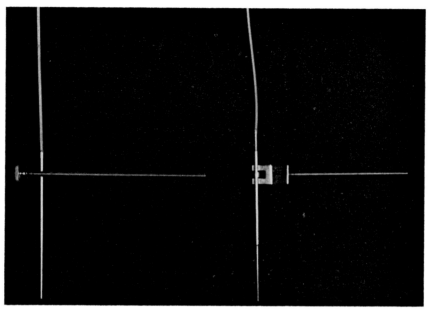

Fig. Intro-7. Sample probes consisting of special aspirating needles and support bars. Model on the left has knurled-head-screw while model on the right has clip for securing needle to bar.

temperature may be set at the conventional temperatures (25-37°C) used in measuring enzyme kinetics.

5. Sensing devices and recorders: Colorimeters, flame photometers and fluorometers are used in the methods described. The colorimeter employs the dual beam principle and registers differences in photocell output from the reference and flow cells. This difference is then traced as per cent transmittance on a conventional chart recorder or may be presented in digital form. The use of a dual beam gives the colorimeter the greater stability usually associated with this principle. The filters supplied with the colorimeter are usually narrow-band-pass interference types. The initial balancing of circuits between reference and sample light sources is accomplished by a selection of manually inserted orifices of different sizes in the light path in combination with a potentiometer. A flame photometer and fluorometers are used similarly. Importantly, the stream of colored, fluorescent, or "burning" solution is "de-bubbled" just prior to passing through the flow-cell or burner.

The micro methods described utilize standard AutoAnalyzer modules and equipment either manufactured or distributed by Technicon Instruments Corp. The new thin Type "C" membrane is used for dialysis, and the 15 mm tubular flow cell is used in the colorimeter. The equipment modifications necessary for performance of the micro-methods are:

Sample probe: A carrier for the aspirating needle was constructed in order that the sample be obtained from the exact center and bottom of each cup. The needle-probe is a No. 22 gauge, 3.5 inch long spinal needle with the finger grip cut off and a short bevel on the aspirating end; it is secured in the end of

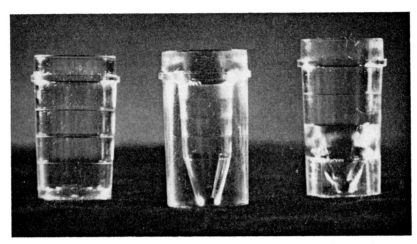

Fig. Intro-8. (Left to right) 2.0 ml. sample cup, new 0.5 ml. sample cup, and 1.5 ml. sample cup.

the crook-holder bar attachment with a hand-tightening knurled-head screw. A "clip" model has been introduced by Technicon®. The needle-probe is connected to the sample pump tube with 0.015 or 0.030 inch internal diameter polyethylene tubing. Polyethylene tubing washes and clears previous samples better than the tygon tubing used throughout the remainder of the systems.

Sample cup: (Technicon Part No. 127093) This new 500 μL capacity sample cup has a narrow internal diameter and conical bottom which provides a low surface-to-volume ratio. The maximum specimen volume of the sealed micro collecting tube is 350 μL and should yield about 150 μL of plasma. This is enough for one group of analyses; care should be taken to fill each sample cup with at least 0.15 ml. of plasma. When venous blood is obtained, larger amounts of the sample may be placed in the specimen cup or in a standard sample cup.

B. *High-Voltage Paper Electrophoresis* (HVPE) is an alternate method for partition and absorption chromatography. It has the advantages of needing little or no preparation of samples, being more rapid, requiring less space, and being more precise than paper chromatography. These factors combine to make tests, traditionally performed by chromatography in research laboratories, suitable for the Central Clinical Laboratory. HVPE equipment may be obtained from several manufacturers or may be constructed in a local machine-electronics shop.

HVPE exploits the differences and degree of ionization between minute quantities of closely-related low-molecular-weight compounds. The charged compound is made to move in an electrical field; these movements are constant for individual compounds under given electrophoretic conditions. Chromatographic location reagents, modified for pH and moisture conditions of the supporting paper, are used. Quantitation is accomplished by direct densitometry. Since the "spots" are in compact bands, the densitometric measurements are relatively precise.

The preparation of the papers for electrophoretic partitioning is greatly en-

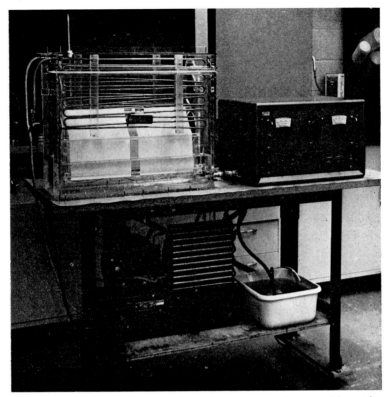

Fig. Intro-9. HVPE apparatus. Tank and power supply on table with cooling unit below.

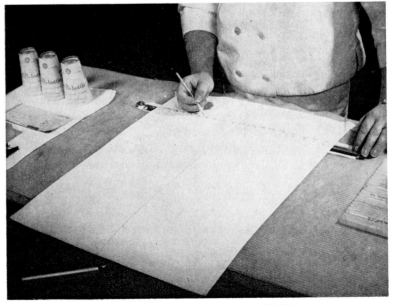

Fig. Intro-10. Technician applying samples to HVPE support paper.

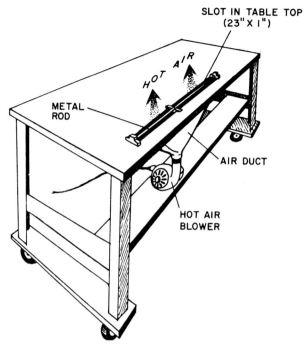

SLOT IN TABLE TOP
(23" X 1")

HOT AIR

METAL
ROD

AIR DUCT

HOT AIR
BLOWER

Fig. Intro-11. Pipetting table.

hanced by use of a pipetting table. The vented slot in the table is designed for drying the application of solutions very rapidly.

QUALITY CONTROL PROCEDURES

The clinical laboratory should provide itself with a system of control which will alert the analyst to any errors. Our laboratory uses the following procedures:

1. Serum pool analysis: All unused patient serum is saved and frozen each day. When a large volume has accumulated, it is thawed and pooled. Then it is divided into ten milliliter aliquots and stored frozen. Each day one sample is thawed and analyzed each time a procedure or test is performed. The values for the control serum are plotted daily on a chart, and analyses are reported for individual patients only if the parallel pool serum analysis is within acceptable control limits.

In order to determine the inherent reproducibility or degree of precision of the method, we calculate the mean and standard deviation for each procedure monthly using the accumulated pool serum test values. First, the average or arithmetic mean is calculated to show the central tendency of the data. This is merely the sum of all values determined divided by the number of determinations. The tendency to dispersion can be expressed as the range from the lowest to the highest values, but a better estimate of the precision of the method can be made by calculating the standard deviation. Standard deviation is a mathematical measure of the dispersion or spread of the data to either side of the mean. Using these data, one can predict that approximately 68 per cent of the values will fall within ±1 standard deviation of the mean, 95 per cent of the values will fall within ±2 standard deviations and 99.7 percent of the values within ±3 standard deviations. Thus, after serum pool values are well-known and the mean and the standard deviations have been established, a serum pool value which deviates from the mean by more than 3 times the standard deviation can be considered "abnormal" or "not due to random errors" since only 3 times in a thousand (0.3 per cent) will the values exceed 3 standard deviations by mere chance.

This same technique may be used to report a variation from the mean of a large number of normal human sera. Thus, a mean value which exceeds more than 3 times the standard deviation may be due to physiological or pathological variation in the patient.

Sometimes it is convenient to express the standard deviation in terms of "per cent of the mean." It is then called the "coefficient of variation."

Example: If a series of determinations gives a mean and standard deviation of 124 and 8.9, then the coefficient of variation would be:

$$\frac{8.9}{124} \times 100 = 7.2\%$$

This system does not measure the accuracy of a determination. It does, however, take into consideration all the variables inherent in a chemical determination such as: (a) reliability of method and reagents, (b) skill of the person or persons performing the test, (c) accuracy and cleanness of pipettes, glassware and cuvets, (d) calibration of colorimeter or spectrophotometer, (e) method used for calculating results, i.e., whether these values were calculated from standards, curves or factors. All of these variables can affect the degree of reproducibility of a particular determination in daily routine work. A sample form to aid in making these calculations is appended.

2. Laboratory inter-comparisons: It is difficult to make comparisons between laboratories because of the use of different procedures and because of the difficulty of transporting specimens without chemical alterations. This is, however, potentially a very important method of control. It is especially convenient for two or three laboratories to serve as a continual check on each other by a system of continuous sample exchange. We accomplish this by periodically including various commercially obtained control sera along with our daily runs.

3. Analysis of known solutions: In most of the methods listed, the use of standard solutions is part of the procedure outlined and is therefore an integral part of the system of control. Another part of this method, when photometric techniques are used, is the maintenance of suitable records so that any untoward variations in the amount of color or emission produced by the standards will at once indicate a problem. This is easily detected in the strip chart recorders. "Weighed in" standards for many metabolites can be obtained from the College of American Pathologists or prepared in the laboratory.

MONTHLY QUALITY CONTROL REPORT

Procedure	1. Average $\overline{X}$ =	Evaluation:
Date	2. Std. Dev. =	
Pool #	# out of control	

Procedure for Calculating Average and
Standard Deviation:

1. Record control analysis in column one.
2. Add column one.
3. Calculate average - line A.
4. Calculate and record in column two individual differences from average.
5. Square each individual difference, and record in column three.
6. Add column three.
7. Calculate standard deviation (SD) - line B.
8. Control limits: $\pm$ 3 x SD = 3 x _____ =

Calculations:

A. x = each individual measurement
    n = number of measurements =

    Average = $\frac{sum\ of\ x}{n}$ or $\frac{x}{n}$

    Average = _____ =

    (Record average in box 1 and 3)

B. Std. Deviation = $\sqrt{\frac{Sum\ of\ squared\ differences\ from\ average}{n\ -\ 1}}$

    Std. Deviation = $\sqrt{}$

    Std. Deviation = $\sqrt{}$

    Std. Deviation =

    (Record in box 2.)

Average: (3)	Diff. from Average:	Squared diff. from Average:
1		
2		
3		
4		
5		
6		
7		
8		
9		
10		
11		
12		
13		
14		
15		
16		
17		
18		
19		
20		
21		
22		
23		
24		
25		
26		
27		
28		
29		
30		
31		

Sum =   Sum of squared difference
                         from average =

To calculate   To calculate standard
the average,   deviation, see line B.
see line A.

Table Intro-1.—Monthly Quality Control Report (Courtesy
American Society of Clinical Pathologists)

4. Blind analysis: Solutions of pure compounds, whose composition is known only to the laboratory director or some other person and not to the analyst, can be a very convenient method of control. If a number of such solutions are prepared, each suitable for several different determinations with different known amounts of substances present, this will prevent conscious or unconscious bias

in the reported results. We participate in one commercially arranged monthly test using this approach.

Thus far we have considered only analytical control and variation. Equally important for interpretation of individual patient results is an awareness of individual and physiological variations. *Individual variation* is the range of values to be expected if the sera of a number of different persons are analyzed. The samples are taken at comparable times to minimize the effect of certain variables mentioned in the next paragraph.

Physiological variation is the range of values to be expected if samples are taken from one individual at various times during the day or night, at various times during his life, or under various types and degrees of physiological stress. Some of these variations are predictable or controllable; others are uncontrollable. They are due to such variables as: sex, age, previous dietary history, body weight and height, mental state, degree of muscle activity, etc.

To minimize some of these variations, blood samples are usually taken with the patient in a fasting or post-prandial state, some 12–14 hours after the last meal. In some cases it is important to avoid exercise prior to blood collection or during a series of blood collections.

REFERENCES

1. Flokstra, J. H., Varley, A. B., and Hagans, J. A.: Reproducibility and accuracy of clinical laboratory determinations. Am. J. Med. Sc. 251: 646–655, 1966.

2. Shively, J. A.: Evaluation of methodology in clinical chemistry. Am. J. Clin. Path. 43: 505–516, 1965.

CHAPTER I

Electrolytes and pH

Clinical Annotation

IN HUMAN PLASMA, as part of the extracellular fluid compartment, the cations sodium and potassium and the anions chloride and bicarbonate are found in greatest concentration. They play important roles controlling osmotic pressure, regulating the exchange of water between the cells of the body, and governing the acid-base equilibrium of the body. Disturbances in the concentrations of these substances are brought about by gastrointestinal losses, abnormal water intake, excess losses via the skin, abnormal electrolyte intake, or inadequate renal or pulmonary function. Even though there are interdependent reactions between these ions, it is difficult and hazardous to predict the changes in one without knowing the changes in the others. For this reason they are usually studied together, which forms the basis for their simultaneous measurement. The concentrations of these ions are expressed in terms of milliequivalents per liter. Associated with abnormal concentrations of plasma electrolytes are disturbances in acid-base equilibirum; these can be monitored by the plasma pH. The normal pH of plasma, the pH at which enzymatic processes of the body can proceed at rates considered normal, is pH 7.35 to 7.45. An increase above 7.45 is alkalosis, and a decrease below 7.35 is acidosis.

Collection Notes

Great emphasis always has been placed on collection of blood for carbon dioxide and pH determination under strict anerobic conditions, endeavoring to prevent loss of carbon dioxide into the atmosphere. Syringes have been oiled and heels and fingers to be bled have been placed under mineral oil. This is not only cumbersome, but it has been shown that mineral oil and other petroleum oils have an affinity for carbon dioxide. To reflect best the *in vivo* electrolyte state the following precautions should be taken:

1. The blood should not be collected or stored under vacuum.

2. Serum or heparinized plasma should be used, since anticoagulants such as potassium oxalate cause water shifts which dilute the plasma fraction.

3. The analyses should be performed promptly.

4. When collecting blood by venipuncture for electrolytes, the patient should not exercise the arm or "make a fist." This may increase the potassium concentration by 1 to 2 mEq./L. The use of a tourniquet may increase the carbon dioxide concentration by 2 to 3 mEq./L.

Free-flowing capillary blood provides satisfactory data if rapidly collected, heparinized, and immediately transported to the laboratory for separation and analysis. If the pH is to be determined, both ends of the capillary must be sealed and the pH measured as soon as possible after the specimen is obtained.

Table I-1. Representative Normal Electrolyte Values for Different Ages.

	Na mEq./L.	K mEq./L.	Cl mEq./L.	CO$_2$ mEq./L.	pH (37°C)
Premature (cord)	132* (116-140)†	6.5 (5.0-10.2)	97 (96-104)	17 (14-22)	7.15-7.35
Premature (48 hour)	140 (128-148)	4.2 (3.0-6.0)	102 (97-110)	22 (18-27)	7.35-7.50
Newborn (cord)	147 (126-166)	7.8 (5.6-12.0)	103 (98-110)	———	———
Newborn (48 hour)	149 (139-162)	5.9 (5.0-7.7)	103 (93-112)	22 (19-27)	7.27-7.47
Infant (1 month)	141 (139-146)	4.0 (4.1-5.3)	105 (95-110)	23 (20-28)	7.35-7.45
Child	141 (138-145)	4.2 (3.5-4.7)	104 (101-108)	22 (18-27)	7.35-7.45
Adult	141 (135-151)	4.5 (3.4-5.6)	104 (98-108)	24 (22-27)	7.35-7.45

*Mean.
†Range.

Interpretation of Results

The terminology relating to the concentration of carbon dioxide in serum or plasma is sometimes confusing and justifies additional discussion. Carbon dioxide is carried in the blood in three forms: (1) bicarbonate, HCO$_3^-$, the main form with small amounts of (2) free carbon dioxide in solution, and (3) carbon dioxide combined with water as carbonic acid, H$_2$CO$_3$. The submicro automated method to be described determines carbonate, bicarbonate, carbonic acid, and physically dissolved carbon dioxide present in the specimen. Thus, total carbon dioxide is measured.

Total carbon dioxide, carbon dioxide content, carbon dioxide combining power, and serum bicarbonate have been used in clinicians' vocabularies without the clear understanding that these terms are not interchangeable. Total carbon dioxide as measured by our method closely represents the buffer space outlined in the Gamblegram.

Since capillary blood is essentially arterial blood, there may be small variations in the values when compared with venous blood values. The greater variations are in pH and carbon dioxide. In general, pH is 0.1 to 0.2 greater and total carbon dioxide concentration is 2 to 4 mEq./L. less in arterial than in venous blood.

MICRO-AUTOMATED SIMULTANEOUS ELECTROLYTES (Na, K, Cl, CO₂)

Principles:

The method simultaneously determines sodium, potassium, chloride, and total carbon dioxide from a plasma or serum sample by using both the diluent and recipient streams. The serum is initially diluted with sulfuric acid solution containing lithium nitrate. The acid liberates carbonate, bicarbonate, and dissolved carbon dioxide from the sample into an air segment free of carbon dioxide. The lithium is used as an internal standard in the measurement of sodium and potassium. The diluted sample passes into the dialyzer and chloride, potassium, sodium, and lithium pass into the recipient stream.

When it leaves the dialyzer, the diluted plasma or serum in the donor stream is mixed with an antifoam agent and then enters a liquid-gas separator; the liquid is discarded and the gas phase, containing carbon dioxide, is aspirated. The gaseous stream then segments a weakly alkaline and buffered phenolphthalein solution. As the gas is absorbed into the solution the pH decreases, resulting in a change in the indicator color. The intensity of color is measured in a flow cuvet at 550 mμ.

The recipient stream from the dialyzer goes to a dual-channel flame photometer for the determination of sodium and potassium. Then this air-segmented stream is resampled and mixed with the chloride color reagent. The developed color is measured at 480 mμ in a flow cuvet.

Preparation of Reagents

1. *Stock Lithium Nitrate*

Lithium nitrate	69.0 Gm.
Sulfuric acid, conc.	106.6 ml.
Distilled water, q.s.	2000.0 ml.

   Place approximately 1000 ml. of distilled water in a 2000 ml. volumetric flask. Slowly add the sulfuric acid. Add the lithium and agitate until completely dissolved. Dilute to volume with distilled water and mix thoroughly. The solution contains 500 mEq./L. of $LiNO_3$ in 2N H_2SO_4.

2. *Working Lithium Nitrate*

Stock lithium nitrate	250 ml.
Distilled water, q.s.	2000 ml.

   Dilute stock lithium nitrate with distilled water. Add 1.0 ml. of Brij.-35° and mix thoroughly. This solution contains 62.5 mEq./L. of $LiNO_3$ in 0.25N H_2SO_4.

3. *1 M Sodium Carbonate*

Sodium carbonate	106 Gm.
Distilled water, q.s.	1000 ml.

4. *1 M Sodium Bicarbonate*

Sodium bicarbonate	84 Gm.
Distilled water, q.s.	1000 ml.

5. *Working Buffer*

1 M sodium carbonate	1 part
1 M sodium bicarbonate	2 parts

6. *Phenolphthalein Indicator*

Phenolphthalein	1 Gm.
Methanol	100 ml.

°Brij.-35 is a polyoxyethelene lauryl alcohol ether and may be obtained from Technicon Instruments Corp., Ardsley, New York.

7. *Working Phenolphthalein Indicator*

Carbonate–bicarbonate buffer	0.42 ml.
Phenolphthalein, 1 per cent	6.50 ml.
Distilled water, q.s.	1000.00 ml.

Invert mix and add 0.5 ml. of Brij.-35; then transfer to an amber CO_2 reagent bottle for use. This reagent is stable for approximately one day.

This reagent should be adjusted so that, with water as a reference, a baseline of 20 per cent T $\pm$ 2 per cent T is achieved and an 80 to 90 per cent T "steady state" with a 40 mEq./L. standard. This allows adequate sensitivity with the other standards.

8. *Chloride Color Reagent*

a. Mercuric thiocyanate	3.0 Gm.
Distilled water, q.s.	1000.0 ml.
b. Mercuric nitrate	68.5 Gm.
Nitric acid, conc.	12.6 Gm. (8.87 ml.)
Distilled water, q.s.	1000.0 ml.
c. Ferric nitrate	202.0 Gm.
Nitric acid, conc.	31.5 Gm. (22.18 ml.)
Distilled water, q.s.	1000.0 ml.

To approximately 1500 ml. of filtered mercuric thiocyanate in a 2 L. flask, add 200 ml. of ferric nitrate solution. Dilute to 2 L. with mercuric thiocyanate. Mix and add 1.26 ml. of mercuric nitrate and again mix. Transfer to chloride reagent bottle for use. Refilter if necessary.

9. *Distilled Water Recipient*

Add 0.5 ml. Brij.-35/L. distilled water.

10. *Anti-Foam Reagent (Acid Diluent)*

Dow Corning Anti-Foam B
Sulfuric acid, conc. sp. gr. 1.84

To approximately 1800 ml. water in a 2000 ml. volumetric flask, add 14.5 ml. conc. sulfuric acid. Add water to the 2000 ml. graduation mark. Now add 2 ml. of the Dow-Corning Anti-Foam B. Invert several times to mix. Anti-Foam B will settle out on standing, therefore, shake thoroughly before use. This solution has a final concentration of 0.25 N sulfuric acid.

11. *Sodium Hydroxide Wash Solution (1N)*

Sodium hydroxide	40 Gm.
Distilled water, q.s.	1000 ml.

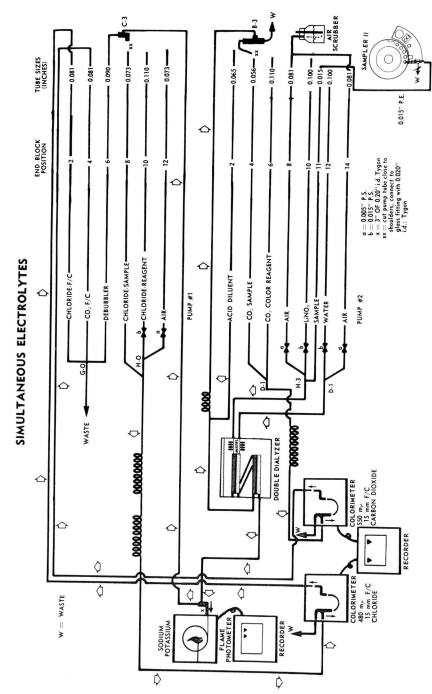

Fig. I-1. Flow diagram for simultaneous electrolytes (Na, K, Cl, CO₂).

12. *Working Standards*

Dilute stock standards (1000 mEq./L.) with distilled water as follows:

No.	ml. Stock Na₂ CO₃	ml. Stock NaCl	ml. Stock KCL	Dilute to
1	40	80	80	1000 ml.
2	30	90	60	1000 ml.
3	20	100	40	1000 ml.
4	10	110	20	1000 ml.
5	—	120	40	1000 ml.
6	—	110	40	1000 ml.
7	—	100	40	1000 ml.
8	30	74	4	1000 ml.

Concentration (mEq./L.) of individual electrolytes in working standards:

No.	mEq. CO_2/L.	mEq. Cl/L.	mEq. Na/L.	mEq. K/L.
1	40	88	160	8
2	30	96	150	6
3	20	104	140	4
4	10	112	130	2
5	—	124	120	4
6	—	114	110	4
7	—	104	100	4
8	30	78	130	4

The standards containing carbonate should not be exposed to air any longer than necessary as they will absorb CO_2 from the atmosphere. They should be stored in 4 oz. bottles that are filled to the brim to exclude air.

Apparatus

The procedure utilizes two proportioning pumps arranged in parallel. The modules used are shown in the flow diagram. For sample line, use 0.015 (ID) polyethylene tubing.

Operating Notes

1. Light flame unit, using the following procedure, 30 minutes prior to run. Remove integrating miror from flame unit and clean with soft cloth.

Turn control knob (potassium channel) to "standby" position. "Flame-out" monitor should sound.

Turn on oxygen by giving main valve wheel at least three complete turns. Main valve gauge should read at least 500 lbs. Second stage gauge should read exactly 50 lbs.

Turn on natural gas by giving main valve wheel at least three complete turns.

Apply lighted match to side of burner unit. Flame should light immediately. Be sure that all three pilots are burning.

2. Turn colorimeters toggle switches to "on" position.

3. Turn recorders to "on" position, but do not turn chart drives on.

4. Pull manifolds to first set of notches in block and start water pumping through system. NOTE: Start both manifolds at same time.

5. Remove "zero" blank from CO_2 colorimeter and adjust to 98 per cent T (with water flowing through cuvet) with vernier dial on CO_2 colorimeter.

6. Aspirate reagents through all lines except CO_2 color reagent line which should pump water. Set CO_2 colorimeter to give 98 per cent T reading with water since this is an inverse color technique.

7. Remove "zero" blank from Cl colorimeter and adjust reagent baseline to 97 to 98 per cent T.

8. Continue pumping reagents until CO_2 recorder pen falls to reagent baseline of 20 to 25 per cent T.

9. Turn potassium channel control knob to "K," indicating channel is open for recording potassium signal.

10. Turn sodium and potassium recorder chart drive on. Pens should move to left, indicating lithium background (baseline).

11. Let entire system run 2 to 3 minutes to be sure of steady baseline.

12. Standards should be placed on the sample tray in the following order: 3 cups of No. 3 followed by 7, 6, 5, 4, 3, 2, 1. The last seven cups will be used to draw the standard curves. Put a No. 3 standard in every tenth cup and fill the remaining cups with unknowns to be analyzed. *Do not leave a blank space in the sampler.*

13. Aspirate No. 1 standard until a "steady state" has been achieved. With calibration controls set both sodium and potassium recorder pens between 85 and 90 per cent T. CO_2 reagent should have a steady state of 80 to 90 per cent T, and the chloride reagent should have a value of 55 to 65 per cent T.

14. Turn on sampler module, and be sure sample probe is properly centered. Samples may now be placed on platter covered while the module is sampling.

15. At end of run, pump distilled water through lines for 8 minutes. See flame photometer manual for cleaning of instrument.

16. "Flame-out" and shut-down procedure. When last sample has been recorded, turn chart drives off and stopcocks to water position. Detach flame line and, by means of a 0.045 manifold tube, aspirate fresh distilled water through flame units for at least 3 minutes or until all traces of lithium color (dark red) has disappeared from flame. Detach tube from flame unit and wait for last remnants of water to be aspirated from unit capillary. Allow flame to run "dry" for 5 to 10 seconds. Turn K channel knob to "standby" position. *Turn gas off first.* Flame should go out immediately. Monitor should sound, then turn off oxygen. When both oxygen gauges fall to zero, turn K channel control knob to "off" position.

Replace "zero" blanks in colorimeters.

When manifolds have been washed clear of reagents, release blocks.

NOTE: Flame line (from manifold) *must* be detached before turning off flame. If, for any reason, the proportioning pump need be stopped, detach flame line *first*. Then attach the 0.045 tube to flame unit and aspirate distilled water until pump is started again.

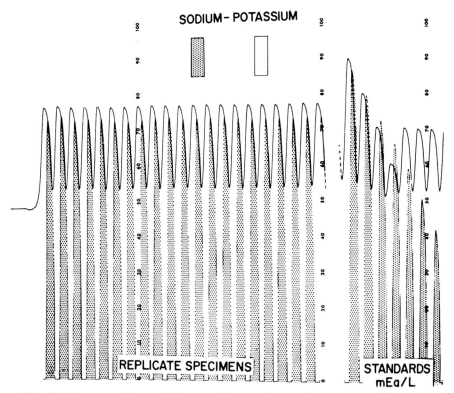

Fig. I-2. Portions of record from sodium and potassium two-pen chart recorder. Sodium standards are 100, 110, 120, 130, 140, 150, and 160 mEq./L. Potassium standards are 2, 4, 6, and 8 mEq./L.

Supplementary Operating Notes

The electrolyte procedure can be run at forty determinations per hour using serum, plasma, spinal fluid or urine samples.

Manifold. The manifold should be constructed as shown in the flow diagram with the pump tubes in the positions shown. Their positions represent the most favorable order and have been designed to prevent overlapping of small pump tubes on the larger ones.

Sodium Hydroxide Wash Bottle. The air which segments the diluent and recipient stream is initially passed through an air scrubber containing 1N sodium hydroxide to remove atmospheric CO_2. The outlet of the air scrubber is also connected to the CO_2 color reagent bottle to prevent exposing the reagent to atmospheric CO_2. The bottle is capped with a two-hole rubber stopper containing a long and a short side arm inserted into the bottle. Both arms extend through the stopper. The short arm extends through the stopper to a level above the sodium hydroxide; it is connected to the air scrubber outlet thus bringing CO_2 free air from the bottle. The long arm extends well below the surface of the sodium hydroxide; it is connected to the air scrubber inlet for entry of room air.

Trouble-Shooting Hints. Be sure to use 0.5 ml. Brij.-35/L. in $LiNO_3$, water

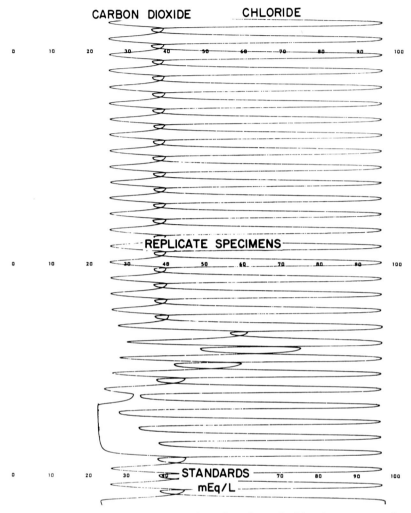

Fig. I-3. Portions of record from carbon dioxide and chloride two-pen chart recorder. Carbon dioxide standards are for 10, 20, 30, and 40 mEq./L. Chloride standards are 78, 88, 96, 104, 112, and 124 mEq./L.

recipient, and CO_2 color reagent for good bubble patterns and low noise levels. If all pump tubes are not pumping evenly, add a helper spring behind center spring at *both* ends of platen. When starting the pump, be sure there is no overlapping of pump tubes under the rollers. If there is, raise rollers and lower again carefully. Tubes which "snake," or show other signs of wear, should be replaced promptly.

Results and Calculations

Calculations of results are obtained by comparing the individual peak heights from a simultaneously prepared standard curve. Cl and CO_2 values are obtained by plotting per cent transmission or optical density of standards versus concentration on graph paper. Na^+ and K^+ values are obtained by plotting per cent transmission of standards versus concentration on regular linear graph paper. In all cases, the per cent transmission obtained for the sample is converted to milli-equivalents per liter by reading the corresponding value from the calibration graph.

SODIUM AND POTASSIUM (Micro Manual)

Principle

Flame photometric analysis (emission photometry) depends upon the fact that when a metal is burned in a flame its molecules are energized and emit a characteristic color. This color may be produced by spraying a solution containing the salt of the metal into the flame. Sodium is identified by a yellow color, potassium produces violet, while lithium imparts a red color to a flame. The intensity of the color is proportional to the amount of the element burned in the flame.

Preparation of Reagents

1. *Lithium Stock*
Lithium Nitrate	5.560 Gm.
Distilled water, q.s.	1000.000 ml.
2. *Lithium Diluent (15 mEq./L. or 104 mg. Li/L.)*
Lithium stock	50.0 ml.
Distilled water, q.s.	200.0 ml.
3. *Standards*
   Same as for automated method.

Apparatus

An International Instrument (IL) Flame Photometer Model #143 is used.

Operating Notes

Make a 1:200 dilution of the sample with the lithium diluent. IMPORTANT: Use same lithium diluent to prepare both standards and unknowns.

Analysis of the Samples

Aspirate lithium diluent through the atomizer of the unit for at least 5 minutes before the calibration procedure is started. Change the lithium solution and aspirate fresh lithium diluent. Set lithium indicator to read in the center of arrowhead. After lithium indicator is set, make both Na and K digital readouts read zero with the zero adjust controls. Lock each control after setting to zero. Remove the lithium stock and insert beaker containing serum or urine standard, whichever is appropriate. Set the "K" range control in the proper position; set the correct values of the standard on both Na and K digital readouts using the appropriate balance controls.

Relace the standard beaker containing the sample correctly diluted with the lithium stock and aspirate the sample. Read the unknowns.

NOTE: Initially, when aspirating unknowns, it is advisable to check the calibration of the instrument after every ten to fifteen samples. Actually, as long as the lithium indicator does not move outside the two lines above or below the arrowhead indicator, drift will be less than 1 mEq./L. of Na and 0.1 mEq./L. of K.

For additional details refer to International Instrument Operating Manual Model #143.

Calculations

The individual sample values are read directly from the individual roller digitals.

CHLORIDE (Micro Manual)

Principle

The theory is based on established principles of coulometric generation of reagent and of amperometric indication of the end point. A constant current is passed between a pair of silver generator electrodes in the generator coulometric circuit, causing release of silver ion into the titration solution at a constant rate. The end point is indicated after all chloride has been precipitated by the increasing concentration of free silver ion which closes a Meter-Relay in the indicator (amperometric) circuit. At a preset increment of indicator current the relay is activated, stopping a timer which runs concurrently with generation of silver ion. Since the rate of generation of silver ion is constant, the amount of chloride precipitated is proportional to the elapsed time.

Preparation of Reagents

1. *Nitric-Acetic Reagent*
   To 1800 ml. of water, add 12.8 ml. concentrated nitric acid and 200 ml. of glacial acetic acid. Mix thoroughly.
2. *Gelatin Reagent*
   To 6.2 Gm. of the supplied dry mixture, add approximately 1 L. of hot water and heat gently with continuous swirling until the solution is clear. Keep in refrigerator, but do not freeze.
3. *Sodium Chloride Standard (100 mEq./L.)*
   Dissolve 5.84 Gm. of oven-dried reagent grade NaCl in water and dilute to 1 L.

Apparatus

Buchler-Cotlove Chloridometer.

Operating Notes

1. Before using this instrument, always clean the electrodes with silver polish.
2. Turn the line switch on and set titration regulator to the "high" position.
3. Set the titrator switch to position #2 and move the adjustable (red)

pointer to the meter relay to coincide with the black indicator to activate the relay which shuts off the titrator (a distinct click will be heard).

4. Allow 5 to 10 minutes for the instrument to warm up.

5. Deliver exactly 4.0 ml. of nitric-acetic diluent into titration vials; two vials for each test; two for the standard and two for a blank.

6. With the Coleman micro pipet deliver exactly 100 lambdas of serum into the vial marked "test," and 100 lambdas of standard (100 mEq./L.) into the vials marked "standard."

7. To all tubes add 4 drops of gelatin reagent.

8. Place the "blank" vial in its fully raised position and turn the titration switch to "adjust" position. The stirrer will start and the indicator pointer will fall within an interval of 10 to 30 seconds to a stable value.

9. Reset timer to zero.

10. Set the adjustable (red) pointer 10 microamperes above the indicator (black) pointer.

11. Turn the titration to the titrate position (#32). The timer will start with the simultaneous generation of silver ions.

12. Record the time required to titrate the sample to the nearest tenth second and average the values for duplicate titration.

13. Remove the vial and rinse electrodes with distilled water.

14. Repeat steps 4 through 10 for the test and standard titrations.

15. For additional details refer to Buchler Instruments instruction manual.

Calculations

$$\frac{\text{Seconds to titrate unknown—blank}}{\text{Seconds to titrate standard—blank}} \times 100 = \text{mEq./L. chlorides of unknown}$$

CARBON DIOXIDE CONTENT (Micro Manual)

Principle

Carbon dioxide is liberated from aqueous solution by lactic acid. The liberated gas is shaken free from the liquid under reduced pressure and then brought to a constant volume to measure pressure (P_1). The CO_2 is absorbed in alkali or otherwise eliminated and the pressure (P_2) of the residual gases measured at the same volume. The pressure drop (P_1–P_2) in millimeters of mercury is multiplied by a temperature-conversion factor to give the CO_2 value at a standard temperature. The volume of liberated gas (CO_2) is, of course, directly proportional to the total carbon dioxide content of the serum or plasma.

Preparation of Reagents

1. *Lactic Acid Solutions*

Lactic acid, 85 per cent	90 ml.
Distilled water, q.s.	1000 ml.

Dilute to 85 per cent lactic acid with distilled water. Transfer 5 ml. of this solution to a vial and add 2 ml. of mercury.

2. *Sodium Hydroxide (3N)*

Sodium hydroxide	12 Gm.
Distilled water, q.s.	100 ml.

Dissolve NaOH in distilled H_2O and dilute to volume. Transfer 5 ml. of this solution to a vial and add 5 ml. of mercury and keep stoppered well.

3. *Low Foam Detergent, 0.5 Per Cent*

Scientific Industries Reagent #810	10 ml.
Distilled water, q.s.	100 ml.

Mix 0.5 per cent low foam detergent and transfer about 5 ml. to a vial and add about 2 ml. of mercury.

4. *Antifoam, 10 Per Cent*

Scientific Industries Reagent #820

Use as purchased. Shake well, transfer about 10 ml. to a vial, and add about 2 ml. of mercury.

Apparatus

A Natelson Microgasometer Model 600 is used.

Operating Notes

1. Start with a drop of mercury on the end of the pipet.
2. Sample—0.03 ml. of specimen and 0.01 to 0.02 ml. of mercury.
3. Lactic acid—0.03 ml. lactic acid and 0.01 to 0.02 ml. mercury.
4. Antifoam—shake before using. 0.01 ml. antifoam and 0.01 to 0.02 ml. mercury.
5. Low-foam detergent—0.1 ml. of low-foam detergent, then mercury to the 0.12 mark of reaction chamber.
6. Close reaction chamber stopcock before taking pipet out of mercury to the 0.12 mark of reaction chamber.
7. Loosen clamping knob and shake for 1 minute.
8. Advance piston until aqueous meniscus is at 0.12.
9. Record manometer reading P_1 and temperature.
10. Advance piston till mercury is at top of manometer.
11. Hold NaOH vial under pipet and open reaction chamber stopcock.
12. Adjust mercury, if necessary, until drop is at tip of pipet.
13. 0.03 ml. of NaOH and mercury to 0.12 mark.
14. Close reaction chamber stopcock and retreat with piston till mercury is at 3 ml. mark. Hold about 5 seconds to permit draining.
15. Advance piston till aqueous meniscus is at 0.12.
16. Record manometer reading P_2'

Calculations

CO_2 content in mEq./L. = $(P_1\text{-}P_2)$ times factor for temperature.

TEMPERATURE FACTORS

17 - 0.242	25 - 0.232
18 - 0.240	26 - 0.231
19 - 0.238	27 - 0.230
20 - 0.237	28 - 0.229
21 - 0.236	29 - 0.228
22 - 0.235	30 - 0.227
23 - 0.234	31 - 0.225
24 - 0.233	32 - 0.224

BLOOD pH

Principle

The pH is a measure of the hydrogen ion concentration. It has been defined as the negative logarithm of the hydrogen ion concentration thus yielding only positive numbers.

Preparation of Reagents

1. pH Reference Buffer Solutions.
    a. pH 7.38, prepared by reputable manufacturer.
    b. pH 6.86, prepared by reputable manufacturer.
    c. Potassium chloride (saturated solution).

Apparatus

A Radiometer pH meter, Type PHM4, is used.

Operating Notes

1. *Battery Test.* Test the batteries by turning the main switch (marked OFF, A, B, C, D, ON) to positions A, B, C, and D, respectively, and make sure that the meter needle rests within the black field of the scale. Then return to "on" position.

2. *Zero Setting.* Set the meter needle to zero by rotating the two "zero" controls, the upper one provides for coarse setting and the lower one for fine setting of the zero.

3. *Standardizing.* Set the "+ / − /pH" range switch to "pH." Readjust the lower "zero" control if required. Set the "temperature" dial to the temperature of the sample (37° C). Press the "standardize" key and adjust the "standardize" controls until the needle is at zero again. Upper knob: Coarse, lower knob; fine. Release the "standardize" key and make sure that the needle remains at zero.

4. *Buffer Adjustment.* Fill the electrode with buffer (pH 7.38) and place it on the support so that the electrode is immersed in the KCl solution. Set the "balance" dials to the pH of the buffer. Reset zero, if required. Press the "balance" button and make sure that the meter indication does not change the instrument and the electrodes are now ready for pH measurements.

5. *Measurement of Whole Blood pH.* Wash the capillary electrode with

saline solution (0.85 per cent). Fill the capillary electrode with heparinized whole blood. Sample should be measured within minutes after being drawn from patient. If measurement is delayed for some reason, insert unopened heparinized blood into ice water or refrigerate (this is not a completely satisfactory procedure).

Place electrode on holder so that salt bridge is closed. Depress "balance" button and rotate "balance" dials until the meter reads zero.

Record the pH.

6. *Cleansing of Electrode.* Rinse electrode with saline. Wash electrode with alternate detergent and air washes. Rinse electrode with distilled water in the capillary.

Calculations

The individual sample value is read directly from the pH meter.

REFERENCES

1. Archarya, P. T., and Payne, W. W.: Blood chemistry of normal full-term infants in the first 48 hours of life. Arch. Dis. Child. 40: 430–435, 1965.

2. Anrode, H. G., and McCrory, W. W.: Comparison of venous and capillary blood electrolyte analysis. Clin. Chem. 2. 278–279, 1956.

3. Bronson, W. R., DeVita, V. T., Carbone, P. P., and Cotlove, E.: Pseudohyperkalemia due to release of potassium from white blood cells during clotting. New Eng. J. Med. 274: 369–375, 1966.

4. Cotlove, E., Trentham, H. V., and Bowman, R. L.: An instrument and method for automatic, rapid, accurate and sensitive titration of chloride in biologic samples. J. Lab. Clin. Med. 51: 461–468, 1958.

5. Mabry, C. C., Gevedon, R. E., Roeckel, I. E., and Gochman, N.: Automated submicrochemistries; A system of rapid sub-microchemical analysis for the measurement of sodium potassium, chloride, carbon dioxide, sugar, urea nitrogen, total and direct reacting bilirubin and total protein. Amer. J. Clin. Path. 46: 265–281, 1966.

6. Oliver, Jr., T. K., Young, G. A., Bates, G. D., and Adams, J. S.: Factitial hyperkalemia due to icing before analysis. Pediatrics. 38: 900–902, 1966.

7. Portnoy, H. D., Thomas, L. M., and Gurdjian, E.: Storage of blood for measurements of pH, PO_2, PCO_2. Clin. Chem. Acta. 11:268–269, 1965.

8. Yu, J., Payne, W. W., Ifekwunigiwe, A., and Stevens, J.: Biochemical status of healthy premature infants in the first 48 hours of life. Arch. Dis. Child. 40: 516–525, 1965.

CHAPTER II

Total Sugar and Protein Metabolites

Clinical Annotation

THE MAIN PHASES of carbohydrate metabolism consist of intestinal digestion of polysaccharides, intestinal absorption of the resultant monosaccharides, their transport to the liver with subsequent anabolism and storage as glycogen, reconversion or mobilization of the glycogen into glucose, its transport to the extrahepatic tissues, and, finally, utilization of the glucose by the tissue cells. Under normal and pathologic conditions, the blood concentration of glucose, from moment to moment, is a reflection of these coordinated and opposing forces. Thus, the measurement of blood sugar, or blood glucose, is important in assessing many pathologic conditions. There are many clinical disorders in which the blood sugar concentration may be greatly altered, especially those involving the islet cells, pituitary and adrenal glands, liver, and intestines.

Urea is a degradation product of protein metabolism and, like blood glucose, the concentration in the serum represents a summation of various metabolic factors included in absorption, turnover, and excretion. Although urea is largely excreted by the glomeruli and regulated by the tubules, increased levels in the plasma offer a crude index of renal impairment, since glomerular destruction must amount to some 80 per cent before urea is retained. Diminished blood urea concentrations are usually a reflection of either impaired intestinal absorption of protein or impaired liver degradation of protein.

Creatine, a methylated amino acid complex, is synthesized in large part in the liver and then is carried to muscle. Creatinine is considered a waste product of muscle metabolism, and it is derived from creatine. Conversion of creatine to cretainine is an irreversible reaction. In adults, small amounts of creatine are present in blood but are normally absent in urine, except for its occasional excretion in women. Children, however, normally excrete creatine in small amounts. Hypercreatinuria occurs in muscle-wasting disorders such as muscular dystrophy, hyperthyroidism, and poliomyelitis. Creatinine is a normal constituent of blood and urine throughout life. It is normally not reabsorbed by the renal tubules, which makes it useful in estimation of glomerular filtration rates.

Uric acid is derived from endogenous and exogenous purine metabolism and degradation. Most purine derivatives are interconverted so that uric acid occurs in significant concentration both in plasma and urine. Hyperuricemia may be due to such diverse factors as impaired renal function, gout, leukemia, and other disorders. One of these is the newly described X-linked hereditary hyperuricemia associated with mental retardation, choreoathetosis, and self mutilation.

Collection Notes

Plasma or serum is suitable for the above metabolites, but serum is less troublesome in that no preservatives are present which might alter the chemical reactions and fibrinous strands that foul pump lines are less apt to occur. Either should be separated from the blood cells promptly because (1) for blood glucose there is up to a 5 per cent per hour disappearance at room temperature due to utilization of glucose by blood cells and (2) for these metabolites there is a disproportion between their erythrocyte and plasma concentrations since erythrocytes are composed of only about two-thirds water.

Interpretation of Results

The conventional reduction methods for blood sugar estimation do not yield identical results because the chemical material actually measured varies with the method used. As determined by any assay measuring total reducing substance, the value obtained consists not only of glucose but also of smaller or larger amounts of so-called saccharoids—that is, non-sugar-reducing substances such as glutathione, thionine, creatine, uric acid, and glucoronic acid. Also, there are trace amounts of monosaccharides and disaccharides other than glucose in serum. The sum of these substances may amount to as much as 25 mg. of glucose equivalents per 100 ml. of normal plasma or serum. Actually, the amount of this residual reduction varies with the method used. For instance, the Folin-Wu method gives values 10 to 15 per cent greater than the actual blood glucose. A closer estimate to blood glucose is that of the Nelson-Somogyi method which removes most of the saccharoids so that the estimation is in the order of 5 mg. per cent greater than true blood glucose. The alkaline ferricyanide method we use gives values intermediate to these methods.

In normal blood, only the glucose level is approximately the same in the erythrocytes and serum or plasma. Non-glucose reduction is mainly of erythrocyte origin, being several times higher in red cells than in serum or plasma. Thus, when using plasma or serum, one measures blood glucose more closely than when using blood sugar methods which measure substances both in the erythrocyte and the plasma. Also, there is a capillary (arterial) and venous difference in glucose concentration. The capillary glucose concentration may be 40 mg./100 ml. greater than the venous concentration at times of hyperglycemia; in the postabsorptive state the difference is only several milligrams per 100 ml. These differences in distribution of blood glucose and saccharoids are of considerable technical interest, but usually do not impair clinical interpretation of results.

The concentrations of urea, creatine, creatinine, and uric acid are not subject to the wide moment-to-moment changes seen with plasma glucose. Urea nitrogen concentrations normally range between 5 and 20 mg./100 ml. For small infants who usually are receiving a high dietary nitrogen load, the plasma or serum urea nitrogen concentration may be greatly elevated. The renal threshold for creatine is a plasma concentration above 0.6 mg./100 ml. When there is impaired glomerular function, creatine concentration in plasma may rise above 18 mg./100 ml. In the presence of elevated plasma creatinine, tubular reabsorption occurs and plasma or serum creatinine levels no longer reflect only glomerular filtration. For uric acid, normal values in children range between 2 and 5 mg./100 ml.

SIMULTANEOUS SUGAR AND UREA NITROGEN

Principles

Reducing sugar is determined by a procedure utilizing the potassium ferricyanide-potassium ferrocyanide oxidation-reduction reaction. The yellow solution of potassium ferricyanide is reduced to the colorless ferrocyanide. The color is measured at 420 mμ using a flowcell.

The urea nitrogen procedure is a modification of the carbaminodiacetyl reaction as applied to the determination of urea nitrogen. It is based on the direct reaction of urea and diacetyl monoxime (2, 3 butanedione-2-oxime) in the presence of thiosemicarbazide under acidic conditions. The presence of thiosemicarbazide intensifies the color of the reaction product and enables the determination to be run without the need of concentrated acid. In acid solution, diacetyl monoxime is hydrolyzed to diacetyl, which reacts directly with urea in the presence of an acidic ferric alum reagent to form triazine derivatives by an oxidative condensation reaction. The color production of the reaction is measured at 520 mμ using a flowcell.

Preparation of Reagents

1. *Sodium Chloride Solution*

Sodium chloride	18 Gm.
Distilled water, q.s.	2000 ml.

Place the sodium chloride in a 2000 ml. volumetric flask and add approximately 1000 ml. of water. Shake the flask until all the sodium chloride is dissolved. Add water to the 2000 ml. graduation mark. Add 1 ml. of Brij.-35, and mix thoroughly. Transfer to the reagent bottle for use.

2. *Urea-N Color Reagent*

   a. *Stock diacetyl monoxime*

Diacetyl monoxime (2,3-butanedione-2-oxime)	50 Gm.
Distilled water, q.s.	2000 ml.

Transfer the diacetyl monoxime to a 2000 ml. volumetric flask and add approximately 1000 ml. water. Place the flask in a container of warm tap water and agitate until all the diacetyl monoxime is dissolved. Add water to the graduation mark and invert several times until the contents are thoroughly mixed. Filter entire contents through a double layer of filter paper (33 cm.). Transfer to amber polyethylene bottle for use and storage.

   b. *Stock Thiosemicarbazide*

Thiosemicarbazide	10 Gm.
Distilled water, q.s.	2000 ml.

Place the thiosemicarbazide in a 2000 ml. volumetric flask and add approximately 1000 ml. water. Stir with magnetic mixer until thiosemicarbazide is dissolved. Add water to graduation mark and invert several times until contents are thoroughly mixed. Filter entire contents through a double layer of filter paper (33 cm.). Transfer to an amber polyethylene bottle for use and storage.

c. *Working Urea-N Color Reagent*

Stock diacetyl monoxime (a)	133 ml.
Stock thiosemicarbazide (b)	133 ml.
Distilled water, q.s.	2000 ml.

To a 2000 ml. volumetric flask containing 500 ml. distilled water add the stock thiosemicarbazide and diacetyl monoxime solutions. Mix well, bring to volume with distilled water and mix. Transfer to amber polyethylene bottle for use and storage. Add 1 ml. Brij.-35 and mix.

3. *Acid for Urea-N Determination*

a. *Stock Ferric Chloride-Phosphoric Acid*

Ferric chloride ($FeCl_3 \cdot 6H_2O$)	30 Gm.
Phosphoric acid (85 per cent)	600 ml.
Distilled water, q.s.	900 ml.

Dissolve ferric chloride in 30 ml. of water. Transfer to a 500 ml. graduated cylinder. Add phosphoric acid slowly, and swirl cylinder. Add distilled water to 450 ml. mark. Transfer to 1000 ml. erlenmeyer flask and mix; transfer to amber polyethylene bottle for use and storage.

b. *Stock Sulfuric Acid (25 Per Cent)*

Concentrated sulfuric acid	500 ml.
Distilled water, q.s.	2000 ml.

To 1000 ml. of distilled water in a 2000 ml. erlenmeyer slowly add sulfuric acid. Mix and cool. Transfer to a 2000 ml. volumetric flask and bring to volume with distilled water.

c. *Working Acid*

Stock ferric chloride-phosphoric acid (a)	2 ml.
Stock 25 per cent sulfuric acid, q.s.	2000 ml.

Place approximately 1000 ml. of stock 25 per cent sulfuric acid in a volumetric flask. Add 2 ml. stock ferric chloride-phosphoric acid and mix. Dilute to volume with stock 25 per cent sulfuric acid and mix. Transfer to polyethylene bottle for use and storage.

4. *Alkaline Potassium Ferricyanide*

Sodium chloride	18.00 Gm.
Potassium ferricyanide	0.38 Gm.
Sodium carbonate (anhydrous)	40.00 Gm.
Distilled water, q.s.	2000.00 ml.

Place approximately 400 ml. of distilled water in a 2000 ml. volumetric flask. Add the sodium chloride and shake until completely dissolved. In a separate container (a small 50 ml. beaker), place the ferricyanide. Add approximately 30 ml. of water and stir until completely dissolved; transfer the dissolved potassium ferricyanide solution to the 2000 ml. flask. Wash the beaker at least three times with small amounts of water, transferring the washings to the 2000 ml. flask. Transfer the sodium carbonate to a 500 ml. beaker; add approximately 300 ml. distilled water. Heat the contents to approximately 60° C. Stir the carbonate until completely dissolved. Wash the beaker with distilled water at least three times, transferring the washings to the 2000 ml. flask. Add the distilled water to the 2000 ml. graduation mark and invert to mix thoroughly, then add 1 ml. Brij.-35 to the flask and mix again. Transfer the contents to a brown Nalgene bottle. Adjust base line with potassium ferricyanide to obtain sensitivity desired.

5. *Stock Standards*
    a. *Stock Glucose, 10 mg./ml.*

Glucose	10 Gm.
Saturated benzoic acid, q.s.	1000 ml.

    b. *Stock Urea Nitrogen, 10 mg./ml.*

Urea C.P., A.C.S.	21.433 Gm.
Sulfuric acid, 0.01 N, q.s.	1000.000 ml.

6. *Working Standards (Combined Glucose and Urea Nitrogen)*

ml. Stock Glucose	ml. Stock Urea Nitrogen	Dilute to:	mg./100 ml. Glucose	mg./100 ml. Urea Nitrogen
5.0	1.0	100 ml.	50	10
10.0	3.0	100 ml.	100	30
15.0	5.0	100 ml.	150	50
20.0	7.0	100 ml.	200	70
22.5	10.0	100 ml.	225	100
25.0	15.0	100 ml.	250	150
30.0	0.0	100 ml.	300	0

Dilute stock glucose and urea nitrogen with saturated benzoic acid in 0.01 N sulfuric acid, as shown.

Apparatus

The procedure employs one basic unit including a heating bath and an extra colorimeter. A two-pen recorder is also employed. The flow diagram is shown.

Operating Notes

1. Turn recorder module to "on" position by moving top toggle switch upward. Do not turn chart drive on.

2. Turn on colorimeters by toggle switches opposite verniers. Let warm up for at least 15 minutes.

3. Stretch manifold blocks to first or second notches and lock pump rollers on platen. Pump distilled water for 10 to 15 minutes.

4. Turn recorder chart drive on by means of lower toggle switch. Adjust recorder pens to 1 per cent T with black dials on colorimeters.

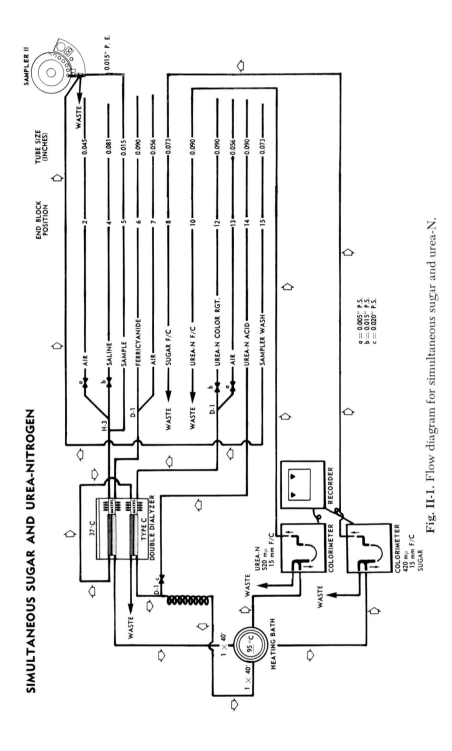

Fig. II-1. Flow diagram for simultaneous sugar and urea-N.

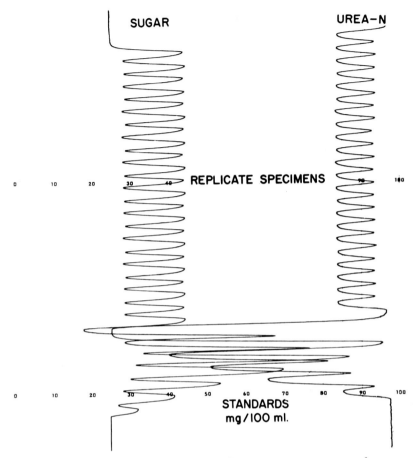

Fig. II-2. Portions of record from sugar and urea nitrogen two-pen chart recorder. Sugar standards are 50, 100, 150, 200, 250, and 300 mg./100 ml. Urea nitrogen standards are 10, 30, 50, 70, 100, and 150 mg./100 ml.

5. Remove "zero" blank from glucose colorimeter and with water pumping through system, adjust, by means of vernier dial on colorimeter, the recorder pen to 99 per cent T.

6. Turn the stopcocks to reagent channels.

7. When glucose recorder pen drops to the ferricyanide baseline, remove the "zero" blank from the BUN colorimeter. Adjust, by means of vernier dial on the BUN colorimeter, the reagent baseline to 98 per cent T.

8. Place standards and samples on the platter. Situate platter on sampler with first standard or sample opposite sampling probe. Keep platter covered during sampling time.

9. When last sample has been recorded, turn off chart drive, replace "zero" blanks in colorimeters, and turn stopcocks to water position. Wash system for at least 10 minutes or until all reagents are washed from the system.

10. Release the rollers and manifold blocks. Leave colorimeters and recorder on during the day.

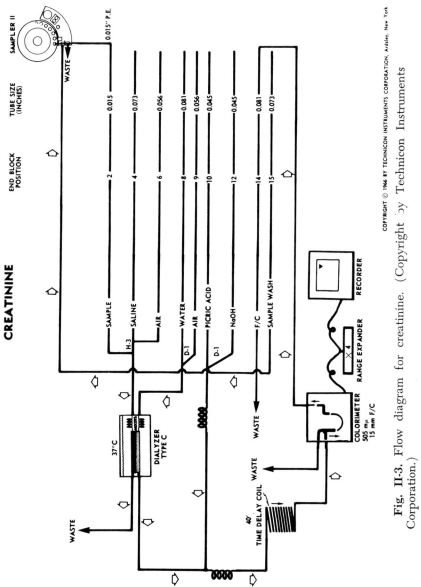

Fig. II-3. Flow diagram for creatinine. (Copyright by Technicon Instruments Corporation.)

11. Run the specimens at the rate of 50/hr.

Calculations

Sample chart recorder tracings are shown. The concentrations are read directly from the chart.

AUTOMATED CREATININE AND CREATINE
(SERUM AND URINE)

Principle

Most of the creatinine methods are dependent upon the Jaffe Reaction, a colorimetric reaction between creatinine and alkaline picrate. In urine, since creatinine is the anhydride of creatine, creatine may be converted to creatinine by boiling (autoclaving) with acid; then its concentration may be determined by the creatinine method. To calculate the creatine, a creatinine determination must be done previous to autoclaving and the differences obtained. This creatinine value is converted to creatine by multiplying by the factor 1.16.

Preparation of Reagents

1. *Isotonic Saline*

Sodium chloride	18 Gm.
Distilled water, q.s.	2000 ml.

Place the sodium chloride in a 2 L. volumetric flask. Add approximately 1000 ml. of distilled water and shake the flask until the sodium chloride is completely dissolved. Dilute to volume and add 1 ml. of Brij.-35.

2. *Sodium Hydroxide*

Sodium hydroxide	40 Gm.
Distilled water, q.s.	2000 ml.

To the sodium hydroxide in a 2 L. volumetric flask add the distilled water. Shake until dissolved and dilute to volume.

3. *Saturated Picric Acid*

Picric acid	26 Gm.
Distilled water, q.s.	2000 ml.

Place the picric acid in a 2 L. volumetric flask. Add about half of the distilled water and shake. Dilute to volume and allow the excess picric acid to remain in contact with the water and shake occasionally. Filter and store in a polyethylene bottle.

4. *Standards*

Creatinine	1 Gm.
Hydrochloric acid, 0.1 N, q.s.	1000 ml.

Weigh out the creatinine on the analytical balance and transfer to a 1 L. volumetric flask. Dissolve and dilute to volume with a 0.1 N HCl.

5. *Working Standards*

ml. of Stock	Dilute to:	mg. Creatinine/100 ml.
1	100 ml.	1
3	100 ml.	3
5	100 ml.	5
7	100 ml.	7
10	100 ml.	10

Dilute the stock creatinine standard with distilled water. Store the dilute standards in the refrigerator.

Apparatus

The procedure employs a basic unit with a time delay coil. The manifold used is shown.

Operating Notes

1. Turn the recorder module to "on" position by moving top toggle switch upward. Do not turn chart drive on.

2. Turn colorimeter on by toggle switch opposite vernier. Let warm up at least 15 minutes.

3. Stretch manifold block to first or second notches and lock pump rollers on the platen. Pump water through system for 10 to 15 minutes.

4. Switch reagent lines on.

5. After about 5 minutes, turn recorder chart drive on by means of lower toggle switch. Adjust the recorder pen to 1 per cent transmission or 0.2 O.D. with black dial on colorimeter.

6. Remove "zero" blank from colorimeter and by means of vernier dial set reagent baseline at 95 to 98 per cent transmission.

7. Place standard and serum samples on platter.* Situate platter on the sampler with first standard or sample opposite sampling probe. Keep platter covered during sampling.

8. Run the specimens at the rate of 40/hr.

9. When last sample has been recorded, turn off the chart drive and replace the "zero" blank in the colorimeter. Place all the reagent lines in distilled water. Wash the system for at least 30 minutes or until all reagents have been washed from the system.

10. Release rollers and manifold block.

Calculations

The results are read directly from the chart recordings. Sample of the tracing is shown.

---

*Creatinine in urine is many times as concentrated as in serum, thus a 1:20 dilution is used. Urine in patients with renal disease may require other dilutions.

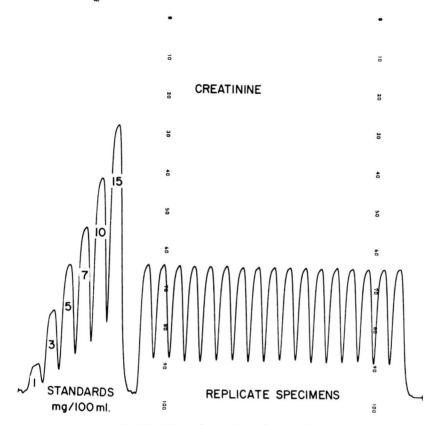

Fig. II-4. Recorder tracing of creatinine.

URIC ACID

Principle

The uric acid determination is based on the ability of uric acid to reduce phosphotungstic acid to yield reduction products which impart a characteristic blue color. The intensity of the blue color is enhanced by a carbonate-urea reagent and is proportional to the amount of uric acid present.

Preparation of Reagents

1. *Isotonic Saline*

Sodium chloride	18 Gm.
Distilled water, q.s.	2000 ml.

Place the sodium chloride in a 2 L. volumetric flask and dilute with water to volume. Add 1 ml. of Aerosol-22 and mix. Filter and store in a 1 L. polyethylene bottle.

2. *Phosphotungstic Acid*

Sodium tungstate	40.0 Gm.
Ortho-phosphoric acid, 85 per cent	32.0 ml.
Lithium sulfate	32.0 Gm.
Distilled water, q.s.	1000.0 ml.

Place the sodium tungstate in a 1 L. flask with a ground glass stopper. Add 300 ml. of distilled water and dissolve the tungstate. Place several glass beads in the flask. Add the 85 per cent ortho-phosphoric acid and mix. Attach a reflux condenser and boil gently for two hours. Cool to room temperature and transfer to a 1 L. volumetric flask. Dilute to volume with water. Add the lithium sulfate and mix well. Filter through filter paper and store in a 1 L. amber bottle. NOTE: The reagent is stable if kept in the refrigerator. Do *not* dilute the phosphotungstic acid.

3. *Cyanide*

Sodium cyanide	100.0 Gm.
Ammonium hydroxide, conc.	2.0 ml.
Distilled water, q.s.	1000.0 ml.

Place the sodium cyanide in a 1 L. volumetric flask and add 950 ml. of distilled water. Mix well and add the ammonium hydroxide and dilute to volume. After mixing well, filter and store in a 1 L. polyethylene bottle.

4. *Urea*

Urea	200.0 Gm.
Distilled water	1000.0 ml.

Place the urea in a 1 L. volumetric flask, dissolve and dilute to volume with water. Filter the solution and store in a polyethylene bottle.

5. *Working Urea-Cyanide Solution*

Stock sodium cyanide	1 part
Stock urea	1 part

Mix this solution on the day before use. NOTE: Label this solution "POISON: DO NOT PIPET BY MOUTH."

6. *Stock Standards*

Uric acid	1.0 Gm.
Lithium carbonate	0.6 Gm.
Formalin, 35 per cent	20.0 ml.
Sulfuric acid, 1 N	25.0 ml.
Distilled water, q.s.	1000.0 ml.

Place the uric acid in a 1 L. volumetric flask. In a separate 250 ml. flask, add the lithium carbonate in 150 ml. of water. Shake 5 minutes until dissolved, then filter off any insoluble material. Heat the warm lithium carbonate solution into the liter volumetric flask while warming it under hot tap water. Shake so as to dissolve the uric acid promptly. In 5 minutes all the uric acid should be dissolved. Shake the flask under cold running water without undue delay. Add the formalin,

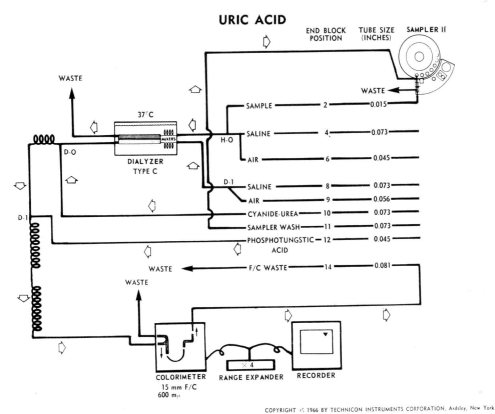

Fig. II-5. Flow diagram for uric acid. (Copyright by Technicon Instruments Corporation.)

and half fill the volumetric flask with distilled water. While shaking slowly add from a pipet 25 ml. of sulfuric acid. Dilute to volume, mix thoroughly, and transfer to a 1 L. amber bottle. This stock solution contains 1 mg. of uric acid per ml.

7. *Working Standards*

ml. of Stock	Dilute to:	mg. Uric Acid per 100 ml.
2	100 ml.	2
4	100 ml.	4
6	100 ml.	6
8	100 ml.	8
10	100 ml.	10

Dilute the stock uric acid standard with distilled water. Store the dilute standards in the refrigerator.

Apparatus

The procedure employs one conventional unit. The manifold used is shown. The interference filter is 660 mμ with a suggested light aperture of 8. For the sample line, use polyethylene, 0.034 × 0.048, tubing.

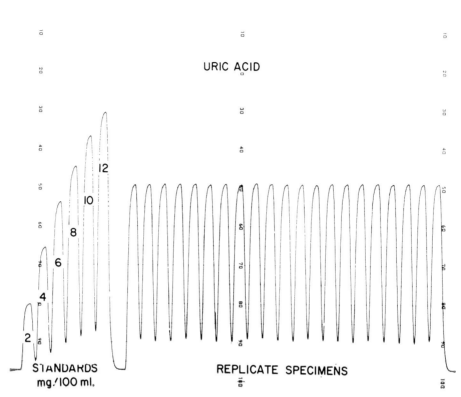

Fig. II-6. Recorder tracing of uric acid.

Operating Notes

1. Turn the recorder module to "on" position by moving top toggle switch upward. Do not turn chart drive on.

2. Turn colorimeter on by toggle switch opposite vernier. Let warm up at least 15 minutes.

3. Stretch manifold block to first or second notches and lock pump rollers on the platen. Pump water through system for 10 to 15 minutes.

4. Switch reagent lines to proper reagent.

5. After about 5 minutes, turn recorder chart drive on by means of lower toggle switch. Adjust the recorder pen to 1 per cent T with black dial on colorimeter.

6. Remove "zero" blank from colorimeter and, by means of vernier dial, set reagent baseline to desired setting.

7. Place standards and samples on platter. Situate platter on the sampler with first standard or sample opposite sampling probe. Keep platter covered during sampling time.

8. Run the specimen at the rate of 40/hr.

9. When last sample has recorded, turn off the chart drive and replace the "zero" blank in the colorimeter. Place all the reagent lines in distilled water.

Wash the system for at least 10 minutes or until all reagents have been washed from the system.

10. Release rollers and manifold block.

Calculations

The results are read directly from the chart recordings. A sample of the tracing is shown.

REFERENCES

1. Cornblath, M., and Reisner, S. H.: Blood glucose in neonate and its clinical significance. New Eng. J. Med. 273: 378–381, 1965.

2. Fingerhut, B., Ferzola, R., Marsh, W. H., and Miller, Jr., A. B.: Automated methods for blood glucose and urea with adaptation for simultaneous determinations. Clin. Chem. 12: 570–576, 1966.

3. Keele, D. K., and Kay, J. L.: Plasma free fatty acid and blood sugar levels in newborn infants and their mothers. Pediatrics. 37: 597–604, 1966.

4. Mabry, C. C., Gevedon, R. E., Roeckel, I. E., and Gochman, N.: Automated submicro-chemistries: A system of rapid submicrochemical analysis for the measurement of sodium, potassium, chloride, carbon dioxide, sugar, urea nitrogen, total and direct-reacting bilirubin and total protein. Amer. J. Clin. Path. 46: 265–281, 1966.

5. Marsh, W. H., Fingerhut, B., and Miller, H.: Automated and manual direct methods for determination of blood urea. Clin. Chem. 11: 624–627, 1965.

6. Moore, J. J., and Sax, S. M.: A revised automated procedure for urea nitrogen. Clin. Chim. Acta. 11: 475–477, 1965.

7. Wybregt, S. H., Reisner, S. H., Patel, R. K., Nellhaus, G., and Cornblath, M.: The incidence of neonatal hypoglycemia in a nursery for premature infants. J. Pediat. 64: 796–802, 1964.

CHAPTER III

Bilirubin and Evaluation of the Jaundiced Infant

Clinical Annotation

BILIRUBIN IS A yellow pigment formed by degrading hemoglobin. Most is derived from erythrocytes at the end of their life span, but a small amount is derived during the synthesis of heme by the immature erythrocyte. It is conjugated with glucoronic acid in the liver, and the product is excreted into the intestine. Normally, a small amount is present in circulating blood tightly bound to albumin, one mole binding two moles of bilirubin. Hyperbilirubinemia, with observable jaundice in the patient, can be caused by excessive hemoglobin breakdown or impairment at any point, either anatomic or physiologic, in the degradation of hemoglobin. Some clinical conditions associated with hyperbilirubinemia are liver disease, obstruction of the bile ducts, hereditary defects in bilirubin conjugation, physiologic jaundice of the newborn which is related to impaired ability to conjugate bilirubin, hemolysis, and sepsis.

The measurement of the degree of hyperbilirubinemia is of special importance in assessing newborn infants with erythroblastosis for the need for exchange transfusion. When the total bilirubin concentration approaches 20 mg. per cent, the intracellular binding forces may be strong enough to compete with albumin binding so that unconjugated bilirubin accumulates within cells where it is potentially toxic. If it accumulates in the basal ganglia of the brain it is called kernicterus, which results in permanent and characteristic neurologic damage. Therefore, the erythroblastotic infant's care is especially dependent on this laboratory measurement.

Collection Notes

The bilirubin content of capillary and venous blood is identical. Care should be exercised to prevent hemolysis, although the method described is affected little by hemolysis. The separated plasma or serum should not be exposed to direct sunlight and should be analyzed promptly. Serum stored in the dark and frozen does not deteriorate over a period of several weeks.

Interpretation of Results

Care must be used in interpreting the cause of hyperbilirubinemia. Usually, a greatly elevated bilirubin concentration, composed mostly of conjugated bilirubin, is associated with anatomic obstruction of the bile flow. Hyperbilirubinemia due to intravascular hemolysis or liver dysfunction is largely unconjugated. So called "physiologic jaundice of the newborn" is frequently associated with a total bilirubin concentration of 12 mg. per cent near the end of the first week of life. We see no justification for diagnosing latent liver

Table III-1. Mechanisms of Persistent Jaundice in Infancy*

Increased Destruction of Red Blood Cells	Liver Parenchyma Injury or Dysfunction	Intrahepatic Biliary Stasis	Extrahepatic Biliary Stasis
Erythroblastosis	Drugs	Drugs	Duodenal atresia
Acquired hemolytic anemias	Cretinism	Cholangitis	Annular pancreas
Autoimmune	Crigler-Najjar disease	Cholestatic jaundice	Pyloric stenosis
DPT immunization	Gilbert's disease		
Favism	Syphilis		Biliary atresia
Drugs	Yellow fever		Choledochal cyst
Primaquine group			Lithiasis
Furadantin group	Leptospirosis		Ascaris or other parasite
Sulfa group	Listeriosis		Local lymphadenopathy
Tetracycline	Herpes simplex		Tumor
Vitamin K	Thyrotoxicosis		
Naphthalene	Transient familial neonatal Hyperbilirubinemia		
Congenital spherocytosis	Pyloric stenosis		
Congenital nonspherocytic anemia	Mongolism		
Hemorrhage with resorption			
Malaria	Physiologic jaundice		
Sickle cell disease	Reticuloendothelioses		
	Septicemia		
	Cytomegalic inclusion disease		
	Galactosemia		
	Toxoplasmosis		
	Neonatal hepatitis or Giant Cell transformation		
	Cirrhosis	Cystic fibrosis	

*Diseases in which jaundice occurs only occasionally or terminally are not listed. Rare diseases which are treatable are included. Extent of crossover between categories is shown by arrows.

Table III-2. Critical Laboratory Tests for Evaluating a Jaundiced Infant

The Infant with Visible Bile in the Stool

1. Hemoglobin, hematocrit
2. Reticulocyte count
3. Morphology of red blood cells
4. Bilirubin, conjugated and unconjugated
5. Glutamic oxaloacetic transaminase, glutamic pyruvic transaminase
6. Cephalin flocculation
7. Set aside acute phase serum to be used subsequently in the study for toxoplasmosis, viral or bacterial diseases
8. Standard test for syphilis
9. Blood culture
10. Reducing substances in urine
11. Inclusion bodies in cells of urine sediment

The Infant with Reduced Amount of Bile in the Stool

1. Hemoglobin, hematocrit
2. Reticulocyte count
3. Glutamic oxaloacetic transaminase, glutamic pyruvic transaminase
4. Serum proteins
5. Serum bilirubin, conjugated and unconjugated
6. Intravenous Rose Bengal-131I with separate 72-hour fecal and urine specimens. If less than 5 per cent of dose is recovered in stool, laparotomy for liver biopsy and exploration of extrahepatic biliary tree is indicated.

disease in nonjaundiced infants who have minor variations in their conjugated bilirubin concentration at a less than 1 mg. per cent level.

AUTOMATED TOTAL AND DIRECT BILIRUBIN

Principle

Quantitative estimation of bilirubin depends on the diazotization of bilirubin to form a colored diazo compound. Serum or plasma is added to a solution of sodium acetate and caffeine-sodium benzoate. The sodium acetate buffers the pH of the diazo reaction, whereas the caffein-sodium benzoate accelerates the coupling of bilirubin with diazotized sulfanilic acid. The azobilirubin color develops rapidly. Ascorbic acid may be used in the total bilirubin measurement to prevent suppression or fading of color intensity by hemoglobin in hemolyzed specimens. Conversion of the neutral-pink azobilirubin to the alkaline-blue azobilirubin for analysis is achieved by adding strong alkali, therefore increasing the specificity by shifting the absorbency maximum to 600 mμ. The final color appears green because blue alkaline azobilirubin is mixed with the yellow pigment derived from the reaction between caffeine and sulfanilic acid. The final color is measured in a 15 mm. flow cell.

Preparation of Reagents

1. *Caffeine Mixture*

Caffeine, purified alkaloid	50.0 Gm.
Sodium benzoate	76.0 Gm.

| Sodium acetate | 126.0 Gm. |
| Distilled water, q.s. | 2000.0 ml. |

Add the above to about 1500 ml. of distilled water and heat to 50° C. When cool, add water to volume. Invert several times to mix and transfer to a 2 L. polyethylene reagent bottle. This reagent is stable for at least six months at room temperature.

2. *Diazo-1*

Sulfanilic acid	10.0 Gm.
Hydrochloric acid, conc.	30.0 ml.
Distilled water, q.s.	2000.0 ml.

Place approximately 1000 ml. of distilled water into a 2 L. volumetric flask. Add the sulfanilic acid and the hydrochloric acid and agitate the flask until the solution is complete. Solution is hastened by using a magnetic stirrer.

3. *Diazo-2*

| Sodium nitrate | 0.5 Gm. |
| Distilled water, q.s. | 100.0 ml. |

Dissolve the sodium nitrate in approximately 75 ml. of water and add the water to the 100 ml. graduation mark. This reagent is stored in a brown bottle at 5° C.

4. *Diazo Reagent*

| Diazo-1 | 200 ml. |
| Diazo-2 | 5 ml. |

This reagent is stable throughout the working day if stored in a brown bottle and shielded from direct light.

5. *Alkaline Mixture*

Sodium hydroxide	50 Gm.
Potassium-sodium tartrate	175 Gm.
Distilled water, q.s.	2000 ml.

Place the above chemicals in approximately 1500 ml. of distilled water in a 2 L. volumetric flask. When all the chemicals have dissolved, dilute to volume with distilled water. This solution is stable for at least six months if stored in a polyethylene bottle.

6. *Ascorbic Acid*

| Ascorbic Acid | 8 Gm. |
| Distilled water, q.s. | 200 ml. |

Dissolve the ascorbic acid in distilled water and dilute to a volume of 200 ml.

CAUTION: This reagent must be made up just before use. Discard any remaining reagent at the end of the day's run.

BILIRUBIN

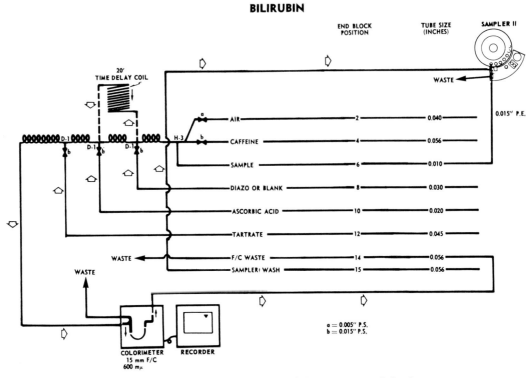

Fig. III-1. Flow diagram for total and direct-reacting bilirubin.

7. 0.05 M Hydrochloric Acid

Hydrochloric acid, conc.	50 ml.
Distilled water, q.s.	1000 ml.

Place about half of the water in a 1 L. volumetric flask and slowly add the acid. Let cool to room temperature and then dilute to volume.

Apparatus

The apparatus and modules needed are outlined on the flow diagram. Sampling is performed at 40/hr.

Preparation of Standards*

The standards are prepared fresh from a commercial "in-serum" laboratory control. This lyophilized sample contains a total bilirubin, almost all unconjugated, of approximately 20 mg./100 ml. when it is reconstituted to 1.0 ml. Six standards, ranging up to the stated value, are prepared by reconstituting the lyophilized control serum with 1 ml., then preparing serial dilutions in separate sample cups. The bilirubin standards and ascorbic acid are prepared fresh for each run.

---

*Acceptable crystalline bilirubin, in chloroform, has a molor absorptivity of 60,700 ± 800 at 453 mμ.

Operating Notes

1. Turn the recorder module to "on" position by moving top toggle switch upward. Do not turn chart drive on.

2. Turn colorimeter on by toggle switch opposite vernier. Let warm up at least 15 minutes.

3. Stretch manifold block to first or second notches, then lock pump rollers on the platen. Pump water through system for 10 to 15 minutes.

4. Switch reagent lines to proper reagents.

5. Pump caffeine, mixed diazo, ascorbic acid and tartrate with delay coil in use for "total" bilirubin.

6. Turn the recorder chart drive on by means of lower toggle switch. Adjust the recorder pen to 1 per cent transmission or 2.0 O.D. with black dial on colorimeter.

7. Remove "zero" blank from colorimeter and, by means of vernier dial, set reagent baseline at 95 to 98 per cent transmission. Continue to pump reagents until a steady baseline is achieved.

8. Place standards and serum samples on platter. *Samples that are frankly icteric are followed by a sample cup of distilled water.* Situate platter on the sampler with first standard opposite sampling probe. Keep platter covered during sampling to exclude light.

9. Aspirate samples at the rate of 40/hr.

10. When last sample has been recorded, rinse the mixed diazo reagent line with distilled water and place in diazo-1 reagent. All other reagents remain the same. Pump this set of reagents until yellow color disappears from final mixing coil on platter. Readjust baseline as for "total" sampling. Resample specimens for "total" blank readings.

11. After the last "total" blank has been recorded, bypass the 20 foot delay coil to a short "1 min." coil for "direct reacting" bilirubin measurements. Also switch caffeine reagent line to 0.05 N HC1 and the diazo-1 line to mixed diazo. Allow these reagents to pump for 10 minutes until a steady baseline is maintained.

12. Sample the specimens a third time for "direct reacting" bilirubin. When the last specimen has been recorded, change mixed diazo line to diazo-1 for the "direct reacting" blanks.

13. After the last sample has been recorded, turn off the chart drive and replace the "zero" blank in the colorimeter. Place all reagent lines in distilled water, and wash for about 30 minutes or until all reagents have been cleared from the system. Remember to wash "total" delay coil.

14. Release rollers and manifold block.

Calculations and Results

The results are read directly from the chart recordings.

MANUAL MICRO TOTAL BILIRUBIN

Principle

Jendrassik-Grof, as described for micro-automated method.

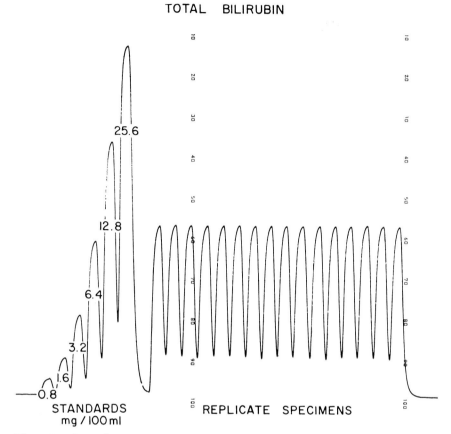

Fig. III-2. Recorder tracing of total bilirubin. Total bilirubin standards are 1 to 25 mg./100 ml.

Preparation of Reagents

1. *Caffeine Mixture*

Caffeine	50 Gm.
Sodium benzoate	75 Gm.
Sodium acetate	126 Gm.
Distilled water, q.s.	1000 ml.

Dissolve the dry reagents in distilled water and dilute to 1 L. volume.

2. *Diazo I*

Sulfanilic acid	5 Gm.
Hydrochloric acid	15 ml.
Distilled water, q.s.	1000 ml.

Dissolve the sulfanilic acid in about 500 ml. of water. Add conc. HCl and dilute to 1 L. volume.

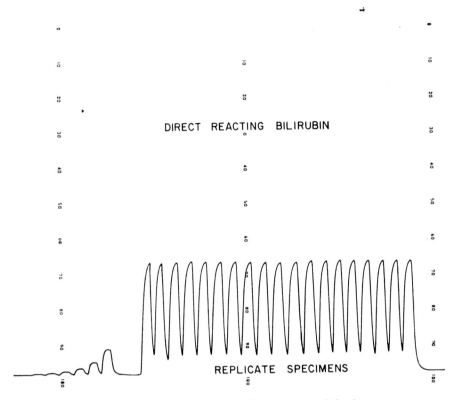

Fig. III-3. Recorder tracing of direct-reacting bilirubin.

3. *Diazo II*

Sodium nitrite   500 mg.
Distilled water, q.s.   100 ml.

Dissolve nitrite in water and dilute to volume of 100 ml. This reagent is stable up to two weeks if stored well stoppered at 4° to 6° C.

4. *Diazo Reagent*

Diazo I   10.00 ml.
Diazo II   0.25 ml.

Add reagents and mix well. Use the reagent within 30 minutes of preparation.

5. *Alkaline Buffer Mixture*

Sodium hydroxide   100 Gm.
Potassium sodium tartrate   350 Gm.
Distilled water, q.s.   1000 ml.

Dissolve dry reagents in water and dilute to volume of 1 L.

6. *Ascorbic Acid, 4 per cent*

    Ascorbic acid   200 mg.

    Distilled water   5 ml.

    Dissolve acid in water and dilute to volume of 5 ml.

Apparatus

Coleman Jr. Spectrophotometer with wavelength set at 600 mμ.

Procedure

Total Bilirubin:	Unknown	Blank
Caffeine mixture	1 ml.	1 ml.
Serum or plasma	50 µL.	50 µL.
Distilled water	.20 ml.	.20 ml.
Diazo reagent (fresh)	250 µL.	250 µL.
Diazo I	—	—
Alkaline mixture	.50 ml.	.50 ml.

Mix caffeine and serum well together. Add water and mix. Add diazo and let stand 10 minutes at room temperature. Add alkaline mixture and mix thoroughly and read within 30 minutes at 600 mμ with blank set at 0 absorbance.

Direct Reacting Bilirubin:	Unknown
0.05 mHCl	1 ml.
Serum or plasma	50 µL.
Distilled water	150 µL.
Diazo reagent (fresh)	250 µL.

Add reagents in order listed, mixing thoroughly after addition of each reagent. Exactly 1 minute after adding the diazo reagent, add 50 lambda of freshly made up ascorbic acid. Mix thoroughly and immediately add 0.5 ml. of alkaline mixture. Mix and read at 600 mμ with blank set at 0 absorbance.

Results and Calculations

The optical density is read directly from the spectrophotometer dial and calculations are made as follows:

$$\frac{\text{O.D. of test}}{\text{O.D. of standard}} \times \text{value of standard} = \text{mg. of bilirubin per 100 ml.}$$

RADIOACTIVE ROSE BENGAL TEST
(for Evaluation of Biliary Patency)

Principle

Rose Bengal is a dye which, when present in circulating plasma, is largely excreted by the liver into the duodenum via the biliary system. Rose Bengal is not significantly reabsorbed by the intestine and thus can be recovered in stool. Rose Bengal labeled with ^{131}I that serves as a marker is used. While in the liver, a portion of the ^{131}I is released from the Rose Bengal molecule; the released ^{131}I is then excreted into the urine or taken up by the thyroid. The longer Rose Bengal remains in the liver, the more ^{131}I is released. In biliary atresia one would expect to recover little or no ^{131}I in stool and large amounts in urine. In hepatocellular dysfunction due to many causes, one would expect to recover some of the marker in stool and excess amounts in urine. In normal individuals, one would expect large amounts of ^{131}I in stool and lesser amounts in urine.

Procedure

1. Administer 2 to 4 drops Lugol's solution orally 6 to 12 hours prior to test to "block" uptake of ^{131}I by thyroid.

2. Feed patient ½ to 1½ hours prior to test to insure maximum biliary function.

3. Apply a urine collection device to males and an indwelling Foley catheter to females.

4. Administer 0.1 μcurie [131]I Rose Bengal per Kg. body weight intravenously by rapid injection. Dilute dose so that at least 2 ml. is administered. At the same time set aside an identical amount of the dose in a plastic container like the one to be used for the separate urine and stool collections. We use 2000 ml. plastic containers.

5. Save all urine and stools separately for 72 hours. It is essential that the urine does not contaminate the stool. Pool the urine and stool specimens separately. No preservatives are required.

Interpretation of Results

	% Dose in 72-hr. Urine	% Dose in 72-hr. Stool
Normal	5-15	40-90
Hepatocellular disease	10-20	10-70
Biliary obstruction	15-25	0-7

REFERENCES

BILIRUBIN

1. Lester, R., and Schmid, R.: Medical progress; Bilirubin metabolism. New Eng. J. Med. 270:779–786, 1964.

2. Mabry, C. C., Gevedon, R. E., Roeckel, I. E., and Gochman, N.: Automated submicrochemistries: A system of rapid submicrochemical analysis for the measurement of sodium potassium, chloride, carbon dioxide, sugar, urea nitrogen, total and direct-reacting bilirubin, and total protein. Amer. J. Clin. Path. 46:265–281, 1966.

3. Sherrick, J. C., and Davis, M. A.: Measurement of serum bilirubin. In Sunderman, F. W. (Ed.): Manual of Procedures for the Applied Seminar on Laboratory Diagnosis of Liver Diseases. Philadelphia, Association of Clinical Scientists, 1966, pp. XII 1–14.

BILIARY PATENCY

1. Brent, R. L., and Geppert, L. J.: The use of radioactive rose bengal in evaluation of infantile jaundice. AMA J. Dis. Child. 98:720–730, 1959.

2. Sharp, H. L., Krivit, W., and Lowman, J. T.: The diagnosis of complete extrahepatic obstruction by Rose Bengal I[131]. J. Pediat. 70:46–53, 1967.

3. White, W. E., Welsh, J. S., Darrow, D. C., and Holder, T. M.: Pediatric application of the radioiodine (I[131]) rose bengal method in hepatic and biliary system disease. Pediatrics. 32:239–250, 1963.

CHAPTER IV

Inorganics

Clinical Annotation

OF THE VARIOUS inorganic substances in plasma, exclusive of the electrolytes described earlier, calcium and phosphorus are found in largest concentration. The normal values vary with age and state of nutrition. When abnormalities occur in the concentration of one, the other usually is reciprocally elevated or depressed. Hypercalcemia is found in idiopathic hypercalcemia, vitamin-D intoxication, hyperparathyroidism and disorders in which the serum protein level is greatly elevated. Hypocalcemia is associated with hypoparathyroidism, secondarily to hyperphosphatemia as in chronic renal failure, in all forms of rickets, in postacidotic states with hypoalbuminemia, and in infantile tetany. Special concern is focused on the serum phosphorus in renal disorders and in associated abnormalities of calcium metabolism.

Magnesium, although found in low concentration in plasma, is an important intracellular ion. The syndrome of magnesium deficiency in man is now well recognized and consists of signs of tetany, convulsion, depression, vertigo, ataxia, muscular weakness and wasting. It occurs in states of protein malnutrition, in primary aldosteronism, and with malabsorption steatorrhea.

Iron is transported in the plasma bound to a specific iron-binding protein, a β-globulin having a molecular weight of about 90,000. Each molecule of this globulin, also known as transferrin or siderophilin, can combine with two atoms of ferric ion. It is presumed that this is a system for the transportation of iron to various areas of the body, since unbound ferric ion is toxic to living tissue. Transferrin gives up the iron to cells for metabolic activity within the cell. In the normal state, about one-third of the iron-binding sites are occupied by iron. The total capacity for iron is called total iron-binding capacity (TIBC), whereas the potential iron-binding capacity is designated the latent or unsaturated iron-binding capacity (LIBC or UIBC).

Although the measurement of serum iron is of primary importance in the assessment of disorders of iron metabolism, the measurement of total iron-binding capacity is of some importance in certain clinical states. For example, in iron deficiency anemia, the serum iron levels are quite low, whereas the total iron-binding capacity is characteristically increased. The reason for this elevation is not known. In hemochromatosis (an inborn error of iron metabolism characterized by increased iron absorption) the total iron-binding capacity may be normal or at times even decreased, while the percentage of saturation with iron of the iron-binding protein approaches 100 per cent. In renal diseases in which the iron-binding protein is lost into the urine, the total iron-binding capacity falls to low levels.

Lithium is a trace element both in plasma and in intracellular water, and

Table IV-1. Normal Values for Calcium and Phosphorus at Different Ages.

	Calcium mg.%	Phosphorus mg.%	Magnesium mg.%	Lithium mEq./L.
Newborns: 1-7 days	7.5-13.9	3.5-8.6	1.4-2.9	———
Infants	10.5-12.0	4.5-6.7	1.2-2.7	———
Children	10.0-11.5	4.5-5.5	1.2-2.6	———
Adults	9.0-11.5	2.5-4.0	1.2-2.6	0.0-0.01

Table IV-2. Normal Values for Iron and Iron Binding Capacity.

Serum iron	85-150 micrograms/100 ml.
Unsaturated iron-binding capacity	275-375 micrograms/100 ml.
Total iron-binding capacity	350-450 micrograms/100 ml.
Percent saturation	20-35%

its newly appreciated clinical importance relates to the treatment of several psychiatric conditions with various lithium salts.

Collection Notes

Plasma or serum is equally suitable for analysis, and usually it is not necessary that the blood be obtained after a fast. For calcium, calcium-binding anticoagulants cannot be used. Hemolyzed specimens may spuriously elevate phosphorus levels. For iron, iron-free syringes and glassware must be used. Thus it is convenient to use plastic syringes, Vacutainer® equipment, and plastic tubes. If the test cannot be run immediately, refrigerator storage of the plasma or serum for up to three days is satisfactory.

Interpretation of Results

Since calcium and phosphorus homeostasis is dependent on the dietary intake of both elements and the functional maturity of several organs, the concentrations vary greatly with age. Also, under normal conditions, about half of serum calcium is bound to plasma protein. In conditions associated with hyperproteinemia, the total serum calcium may be greatly elevated whereas the unbound fraction, which is available for physiologic processes, may be present in normal concentration.

The main factors affecting the reliability of serum iron transferrin data are hemolysis, lipemia, ferritin, very high serum iron with low iron-binding capacity, and the presence of circulating synthetic iron complexes such as therapeutic iron saccharates.

Hemolysis affects the serum iron method presented only to a minimal degree; therefore, hemolyzed specimens need not be rejected. Parenterally administered iron may circulate in the plasma for days and cause as yet unsolved difficulties in the serum determination of transferrin-bound iron and total iron-binding capacity. The latter is dependent upon the former measurement. In such cases, the total iron-binding capacity determination using a quantitative immunologic procedure may be useful. In addition, a number of investigators have shown a diurnal variation of serum iron so that the concentration is greatest in the early morning and least in the afternoon. Total iron-binding capacity does not vary diurnally.

CALCIUM

Principle

The purple dye Corinth Ca (disodium-1-hydroxy-4-chloro-2, 2-diazobenzene-1, 8-hydroxy-naphthalene-3, 6-disulfonic acid) becomes red in the presence of calcium. Magnesium and phosphorus normally present in serum do not interfere if the reaction is carried out in a strong alkaline solution. The color change, a decrease in optical density at 620 mμ, is measured using a 15 mm. flow cell with greatly diminished reference light. The degree of color change is proportional to the concentration of calcium in serum or plasma.

Preparation of Reagents

1. *Stock Corinth Ca (2 mg./ml.)*

Corinth Ca	500.00 mg.
Hydrochloric acid, 0.1N	0.75 ml.
Distilled water, q.s.	250.00 ml.

    Put 500 mg. Corinth Ca (Clinton Laboratories, Los Angeles, California) in a 250 ml. volumetric flask and add approximately 200 ml. of distilled water and the HCl. Stir on a magnetic stirrer until dye is competely in solution. Add distilled water to volume and mix thoroughly. If stored in an amber bottle, this solution is stable for at least one month at room temperature.

2. *Working Corinth Ca Solution (0.2 mg./ml.)*

Stock Corinth Ca	10 ml.
Distilled water, q.s.	100 ml.

    Transfer stock Corinth Ca to a 100 ml. volumetric flask. Dilute to volume with distilled water and mix thoroughly. If stored in an amber bottle, this solution is stable for one week.

3. *Sample Diluent*

Sodium chloride	9.0 Gm.
Citric acid	0.5 Gm.
Distilled water, q.s.	1000.0 ml.
ARW-7°	10.0 ml.

    Put the NaCl and $H_3C_6H_5O_7 \cdot H_2O$ in a 1 L. volumetric flask. Add approximately 800 ml. of water. When salts are completely in solution, add ARW-7 and dilute to volume with distilled water. Mix thoroughly.

4. *Alkali Maintenance Solution (5N NaOH)*

Sodium hydroxide	200.0 Gm.
Distilled water, q.s.	1000.0 ml.
ARW-7	0.5 ml.

°ARW-7 is a wetting agent available from Technicon Instruments Corp., Ardsley, New York.

CALCIUM

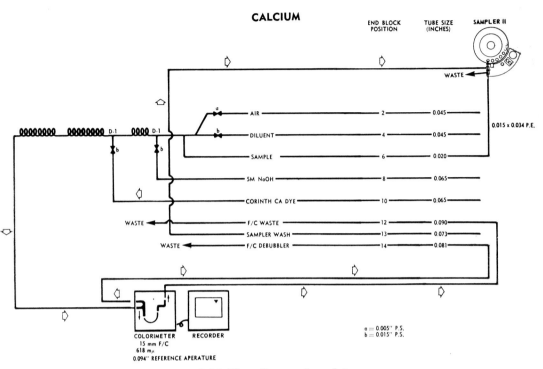

Fig. IV-1. Flow diagram for calcium.

Add NaOH in a 1 L. volumetric flask. Add approximately 800 ml. of distilled water and agitate flask until solution is complete. When flask has cooled to room temperature, add 0.5 ml. of ARW-7 and dilute to volume with distilled water. Mix thoroughly.

5. *Stock Calcium Standard (1 mg. Ca/ml.)*

Calcium carbonate	2.5 Gm.
Hydrochloric acid, conc.	5.0 ml.
Distilled water, q.s.	1000.0 ml.

Place $CaCO_3$ in a 1 L. volumetric flask with approximately 500 ml. of water. Add approximately 5 or 6 ml. of HCl to dissolve the calcium salt. Dilute to volume with distilled water and mix thoroughly.

6. *Working Standards*

These standards are prepared as shown:

ml. of Stock Standard	Using Distilled Water, Dilute to:	Ca^{++} mg. %	Ca^{++} mEq./L.
4.0	100 ml.	4.0	2.0
6.0	100 ml.	6.0	3.0
8.0	100 ml.	8.0	4.0
10.0	100 ml.	10.0	5.0
12.0	100 ml.	12.0	6.0
14.0	100 ml.	14.0	7.0
16.0	100 ml.	16.0	8.0

Apparatus

The equipment used is shown in the flow diagram.

Operating Notes

1. Turn the recorder module to "on" position by moving top toggle switch upward. Do not turn chart drive on.

2. Turn colorimeter on by toggle switch opposite vernier. Let warm up at least 15 minutes.

3. Stretch manifold block to first or second notches and lock pump rollers on the platen. Pump water through system for 10 to 15 minutes.

4. Switch reagent lines to proper reagent except with the working-dye tube pumping water.

5. Remove "zero" blank from colorimeter.

6. After about 5 minutes, turn recorder chart drive on by means of lower toggle switch. Adjust the recorder pens to 1 per cent transmission or 0.01 O.D. with black dial on colorimeter.

7. The dye tube is then placed into the working dye reagent. When the alkaline dye solution reaches the colorimeter cuvet, the recorder pen will move to approximately 1.5 O.D. This is made possible by using a small reference aperature, since the absorbance of the alkali solution is very high. The pen is then shifted downward by the vernier on the colorimeter until the base line is approximately 0.7 O.D. Since absorbancy decreases as the dye complexes with ascending values of calcium, the colorimeter output should drive the recorder pen to approximately 0.05 O.D for the most concentrated (16 mg./100 ml.) standard.

8. Place the standards on the sample platter in ascending order. Follow immediately with the unknown samples. Then situate platter on the sampler with first standard opposite sampling probe. Keep platter covered during sampling. For best quality control, place a serum of known value following every tenth unknown sample.

9. Run specimens at rate of 40/hr.

10. When last sample has been recorded, turn off chart drive and replace "zero" blank in the colorimeter. Place all the reagent lines in distilled water. Wash the system for at least 10 minutes or until all reagents have been washed from the system. For washing, the dye tube should be placed in a separate flask; there is a possibility of contaminating the dye with base if all reagent lines are washed in a common container.

11. Release rollers and manifold block.

12. Should a "noise" level greater than 0.5 per cent develop in this system, the difficulty usually can be traced to poor proportioning of the dye through the D-1 arm of the single mixing coil. This can be corrected by checking all connections and, if necessary, replacing the 0.015 in. pulse suppressor. The viscosity of the 5N NaOH may cause some difficulty, however, the use of the 0.015 in. pulse suppressor and frequent replacement of the NaOH manifold tube should maintain noise-free baselines and peaks.

13. Do not add more wetting agent than specified as excessive amounts of the wetting agent will precipitate upon addition of a strongly alkaline solution.

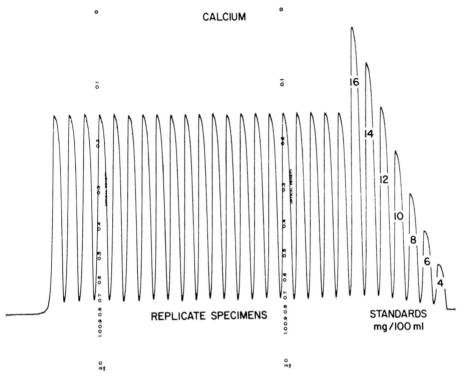

Fig. IV-2. Recorder tracing of calcium.

14. Addendum for Smaller Samples: In the procedure just described, 0.016 ml. of sample is aspirated using the 40 per hour Sampler II cam. Wash between samples is almost complete as shown in the recorder tracing. A smaller sample volume, 0.10 ml., may be aspirated by using a smaller diameter reference aperature (0.625 in.) and a 60 per hour Sampler II cam. The recorder tracings obtained with this smaller sample span the recorder scale as with the larger sample method, but the wash between specimens is not as complete. Nevertheless, the smaller sample is suitable for regular use; carry over between specimens is not significant.

The special reference aperatures used in this method may be made from thin opaque metal or plastic by drilling the appropriate sized hole (6/64 in. or 4/64 in.) in the mid-line two inches from one end of a 1 in. × 3-⅜ in. rectangle.

Results and Calculations

The results are read directly from the chart recordings. A sample tracing is shown.

INORGANIC PHOSPHATE

Principle

The determination of serum or plasma inorganic phosphate depends upon the conversion of inorganic phosphate in a protein free medium to phosphomolybdic acid and the subsequent reduction of this acid to produce a blue color. The reducing agent is stannous chloride-hydrazine sulfate.

Preparation of Reagents

1. *Sulfuric Acid, 10 N*

Sulfuric acid, conc.	278 ml.
Distilled water	1000 ml.

   Slowly add conc. H_2SO_4 to about 500 ml. of water with constant stirring. After cooling, the solution is diluted to 1 L. Subsequent dilutions are made as needed. This method is very sensitive to acid concentration and a wide degree of sensitivity can be achieved by varying the acid concentration in this reagent.

2. *Stannous Chloride-Hydrazine Sulfate Reagent*

Stannous chloride	0.3 Gm.
Hydrazine sulfate	3.0 Gm.
Sulfuric acid, 2N, q.s.	1000.0 ml.

   Dissolve the $SnCl_2 \cdot 2H_2O$ and $H_2NNH_2 \cdot H_2SO_4$ in sulfuric acid and dilute to final volume of 1 L. The resulting solution is stored immediately in a glass-stoppered dark brown bottle at 5° C. A slight precipitate settles slowly on standing, but this does not interfere with the effectiveness of the reagent until after thirty to forty-five days.

3. *Acid Molybdate (7.5 Per Cent in 5N H_2SO_4)*

Sodium molybdate	75 Gm.
Sulfuric acid, 5N	1000 ml.

   Dissolve sodium molybdate in sulfuric acid and dilute to 1 L. volume with 5N H_2SO_4.

4. *Standards*

Inorganic phosphate stock standard (1 mg.P/ml.)	
Potassium phosphate	4.38 Gm.
Distilled water	1000.00 ml.

   Dissolve phosphate in water and dilute to volume of 1 L. Prepare working standards so values will be 1, 3, 5, 7, 10, and 15 mg./100 ml.

Apparatus

The equipment used is shown in the flow diagram.

Operating Notes

1. Turn the recorder module to "on" position by moving top toggle switch upward. Do not turn chart drive on.

2. Turn colorimeter on by toggle switch opposite vernier. Let warm up at least 15 minutes.

3. Stretch manifold block to first or second notches and lock pump rolls on the platen. Pump water through system for 10 to 15 minutes.

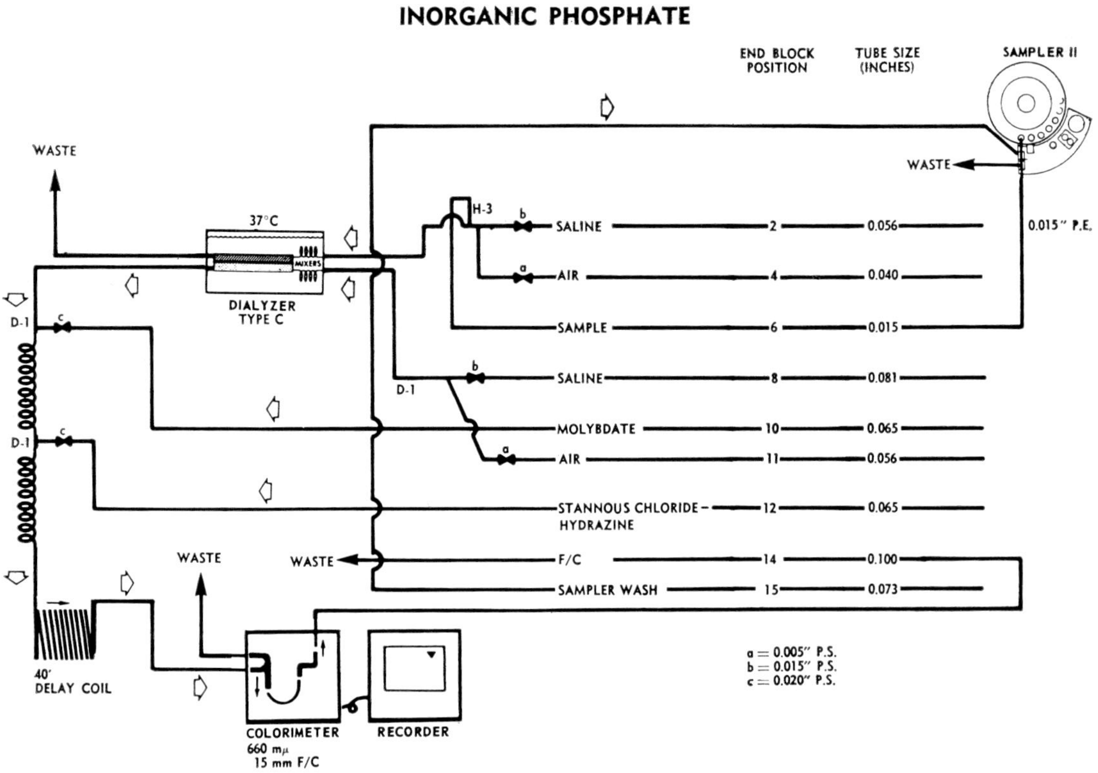

INORGANIC PHOSPHATE

Fig. IV-3. Flow diagram for phosphorus.

4. Switch reagent lines to proper reagents.

5. After about 5 minutes, turn recorder chart drive on by means of lower toggle switch. Adjust the recorder pen to 1 per cent transmission or 0.01 O.D. with black dial on colorimeter.

6. Remove "zero" blank from colorimeter and, by means of vernier dial, set reagent base line to desired setting.

7. Place standard and samples on platter. Situate platter on the sampler with first standard or sample opposite sampling probe. Keep platter covered during sampling. Specimens aspirated are 0.05 ml. in volume.

8. Run the specimens at the rate of 40/hr.

9. When last sample has been recorded, turn off chart drive and replace "zero" blank in the colorimeter. Place all the reagent lines in distilled water. Wash the system for at least 10 minutes or until all reagents have been washed from the system.

10. Release rollers and manifold block.

Results and Calculations

The results are read directly from the chart recordings. A sample of the tracing is shown.

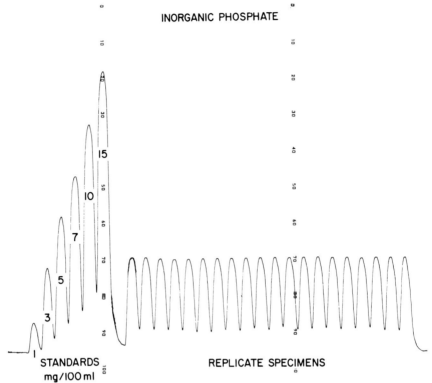

INORGANIC PHOSPHATE

STANDARDS
mg/100 ml

REPLICATE SPECIMENS

Fig. IV-4. Recorder tracing of phosphorus.

MAGNESIUM (Micro Automated)

Principle

A fluorescent complex is produced when magnesium is added to an appropriately buffered and diluted solution of o,ó -dihydroxyazobenzene (o-azophenol). Other cations do not interfere significantly under these conditions. The complex is activated at 470mμ, and the fluorescence is measured at 580 mμ. The intensity of the fluorescence is proportional to the concentration of magnesium.

Preparation of Reagents

1. *Ethylenediamine Solution*

Ethylenediamine, anhydrous	67.0 ml.
Hydrochloric acid, conc.	41.5 ml.
Distilled water, q.s.	500.0 ml.
Ethanol, 95 per cent	500.0 ml.

Add ethylenediamine to approximately 150 ml. of water and mix under a hood. In a separate container, mix the HCl in approximately 150 ml. of water. Under a hood, slowly add the diluted HCl to the diluted ethylenediamine while it is stirred constantly and held under running tap water. Dilute to 500 ml. volume with distilled water, then add 500 ml. of 95 per cent ethanol and mix thoroughly.

2. *Potassium Chloride, 0.34 M*

Potassium chloride	25.0 Gm.
Distilled water	500.0 ml.
Ethanol, 95 per cent	500.0 ml.

Dissolve the KCl in distilled water. Then add 500 ml. 95 percent ethanol. Mix thoroughly.

3. *o-azophenol, 0.125 mM (o,ó -dihydroxyazobenzene)*

o-azophenol	32.5 mg.
Ethanol, 95 per cent	500.0 ml.
Distilled water	500.0 ml.

Dissolve the o-azophenol in the ethanol. Allow to pass through filter paper rapidly and add 500 ml. of water. Mix thoroughly and store in a dark brown glass bottle in the refrigerator. Allow to warm to room temperature before use.

4. *Stock Magnesium Standard*

Magnesium iodate	4.4626 Gm.
Distilled water, q.s.	100.0000 ml.

Dissolve the Mg. $(IO_3)_2$ • $4H_2O$ in distilled water and dilute to volume.

5. *Working Magnesium Standards*

Into 100 ml. volumetric flasks add 0.5 ml., 1.0 ml., 1.5 ml., and 2.0 ml. of stock Mg. standard. Dilute to volume with distilled water, and the Mg. standard values are 1.2, 2.4, 3.6, and 4.8 mg./100 ml., respectively.

Apparatus

The equipment used is shown in the flow diagram.

Operating Notes

1. Turn the recorder module to "on" position by moving top toggle switch upward. Do not turn chart drive on.

2. Turn fluorometer on by toggle switch. After about 2 minutes, press lamp button. Let warm up at least 15 minutes.

3. Stretch manifold block to first or second notches and lock rollers on platen. Pump water through system for 10 to 15 minutes.

4. Switch reagent lines to proper reagents.

5. After about 5 minutes, turn recorder chart drive on by means of lower toggle switch. Adjust the recorder pen to 3 to 5 per cent transmission or about 2.0 O.D. with blank "wheel."

6. Using the range expander, set the high (4.8 mg./100 ml.) standard between 85 and 95 per cent transmission.

7. Place standard and samples on platter. Situate platter on the sampler with first standard or sample opposite sampling probe. Following low to high standards, sample, specimens without introducing an air or water blank. Keep platter covered during sampling. Sample volume is less than 0.05 ml.

MAGNESIUM

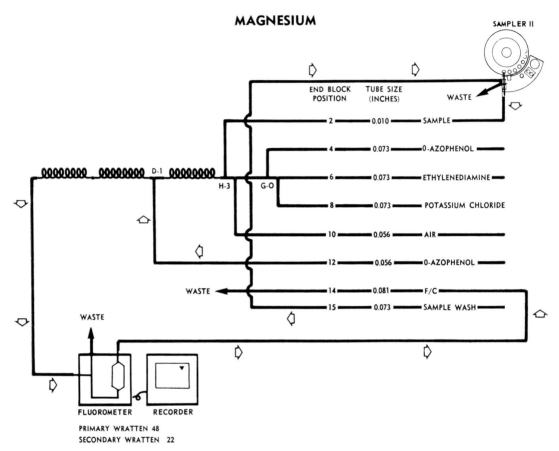

Fig. IV-5. Flow diagram for magnesium.

8. Run at the rate of 50 samples/hr.

9. When last sample has been recorded, turn off chart drive and fluorometer. Place all the reagent lines in distilled water. Wash the system for at least 10 minutes or until all reagents have been washed from the system.

10. Release rollers and manifold block.

Results and Calculations

The results are read directly from the chart recordings. A sample of a tracing is shown.

MAGNESIUM (Micro-Manual)

Principle

Sodium 1-azo-2-hydroxy-3-(2,4 dimethylcarboxanilido)-naphthalene-1-(2-hydroxybenzene-4-sulfonate) at a pH range of 8 to 11 in the presence of magnesium ions changes color from blue-violet to red. The maximum absorb-

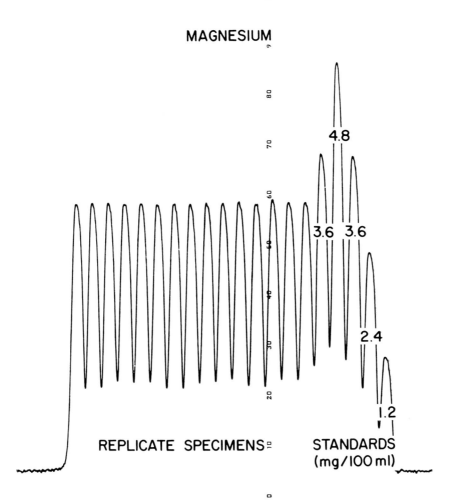

Fig. IV-6. Recorder tracing for magnesium.

ances of the dye reagent and dye reagent-magnesium complex are 555 mμ and 540 mμ, respectively.

Preparation of Reagents

1. *Color Reagent*

1-azo-2-hydroxy-3-(2,4 dimethylcarboxanilido)-naphthalene-1-(2-hydroxybenzene-4-sulfonate) sodium	25 mg.
Absolute alcohol	200 ml.
Distilled water, q.s.	250 ml.

*This reagent may be purchased from LaMotte Chemical Products, Chestertown, Maryland.

Dissolve dry chemical in the absolute alcohol, then dilute to 250 ml. with distilled water.

2. *Sodium Borate Buffer (0.08M)*

Sodium borate	30.51 Gm.
Distilled water, q.s.	1000.00 ml.

Dissolve the sodium borate in approximately 500 ml. of hot distilled water. After cooling to room temperature, dilute the contents to a final volume of 1 L.

3. *Absolute Ethanol*

4. *Magnesium Stock Standard (100 mcgm per ml.)*

Magnesium sulfate	1.0131 Gm.
Distilled water, q.s.	1000.00 ml.

Dissolve the $MgSO_4 \cdot 7H_2O$ in distilled water and dilute to a final volume of 1 L.

5. *Magnesium Working Standard (mcgm per ml.)*

Magnesium stock	1 ml.
Distilled water, q.s.	100 ml.

Dilute stock standard to 100 ml. with distilled water and mix.

Apparatus

A spectrophotometer is used to read the color development.

Operating Notes

1. Into appropriately labeled 25 ml. volumetric flask, measure the following in the order listed:

	Blank	Standards			Control	Unknown
		2 mg.%	4 mg.%	6 mg.%		
Distilled water	10.0 ml.	8.0 ml.	6.0 ml.	4.0 ml.	9.9 ml.	9.9 ml.
Working standards	——	2.0 ml.	4.0 ml.	6.0 ml.	——	——
Harleco control	——	——	——	——	0.1 ml.	——
Unknown serum	——	——	——	——	——	0.1 ml.

2. Add 5.0 ml. of color reagent to each flask and mix.

3. Add 2.0 ml. of borate buffer to all flasks and mix.

4. Dilute all of the flasks to volume with absolute alcohol and allow color to develop for minimum period of 20 minutes. The color is stable up to 24 hours.

5. Measure optical density at 505 mμ in a Coleman Junior Spectrophotometer using 19 mm. cuvets. The reagent blank is used to zero instrument.

Results and Calculations

Calculate magnesium values by plotting standard curve; optical density on the ordinate, and magnesium concentration on abscissa. Then compare the readings of unknowns with the standard curve. An alternate method is by direct calculation using the standard optical density nearest that of the unknown specimen optical density.

$$\frac{\text{O.D. unknown}}{\text{O.D. standard}} \times \text{conc. of standard} = \text{magnesium concentration of unknown.}$$

To convert magnesium values in mg. per cent to mEq./L., divide the value by 1.216.

IRON (Micro-Automated)

Principle

Iron is released from transferrin by hydrochloric acid and reduced by ascorbic acid. It is separated from plasma and serum proteins by dialysis. The free reduced iron is allowed to react with tripyridyl-s-triazine (TPTZ). The intensity of the blue complex formed in a mildly acidic medium is measured at 600 mμ.

Preparation of Reagents

1. *Ascorbic Acid (1 Per Cent w/v)*

Ascorbic acid	1 Gm.
Hydrochloric acid, 1 N	100 ml.

   Place the $C_6H_8O_6$ in a 100 ml. volumetric flask. Add approximately 80 ml. of 1N HCl. Mix until dissolved, then dilute to volume with 1N HCl. Add 2 drops of Brij.-35 and mix thoroughly. Prepare fresh before use.

2. *2, 4, 6-Tripyridyl-1, 3, 5, Triazine (TPTZ)*

2, 4, 6 Tripyridyl-1, 3, 5 triazine	10 mg.
Hydrochloric acid, 1N	100 ml.

   Place the TPTZ in a 100 ml. volumetric flask. Add approximately 80 ml. of 1N HCl. Mix until dissolved, then dilute to volume with 1N HCl. Add 1 drop of Brij.-35 and mix thoroughly.

3. *Ammonium Acetate Solution (5 Per Cent w/v)*

Ammonium acetate	5 Gm.
Distilled water, q.s.	100 ml.

   Place the $NH_4C_2H_3O_2$ in a 100 ml. volumetric flask. Add approximately 80 ml. of distilled water. Mix until dissolved and dilute to volume.

4. *Stock Iron Standard (0.1 mg. Fe/ml.)*

Iron wire, analytical grade	100 mg.
Hydrochloric acid, conc.	20 ml.
Distilled water, q.s.	1000 ml.

   Place the iron wire ni a 500 ml. beaker. Heat the added conc. HCl and approximately 100 ml. of distilled water on a hot plate until solution is complete. A small residue of carbon particles usually

IRON

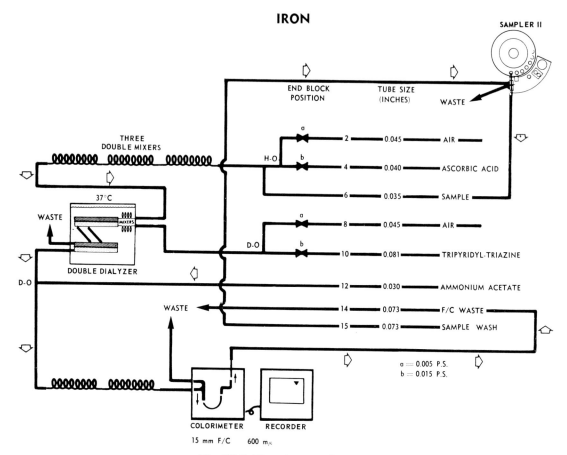

Fig. IV-7. Flow diagram for iron.

remains. Cool the mixture to room temperature, carefully transfer to a 1 L. volumetric flask, and dilute to volume with distilled water.

5. *Working Standard Solutions*

Into 100 ml. volumetric flasks, place 0.5 ml., 1 ml., 2 ml., 3 ml., and 5 ml. of stock iron standard. Dilute to volume with 0.01 N HCl, and the iron standard values are 50, 100, 200, 300, and 500 mg./100 ml., respectively.

6. *Distilled Water*

Double or triple distilled water is suitable for use in this procedure.

Apparatus

The equipment used is shown in the flow diagram.

Operating Notes

1. Turn the recorder module to "on" position by moving top toggle switch upward. Do not turn chart drive on.

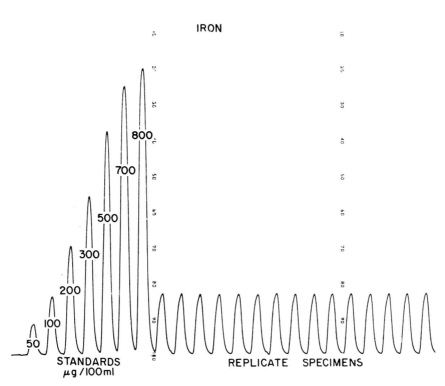

Fig. IV-8. Recorder tracing for iron.

2. Turn colorimeter on by toggle switch opposite vernier. Let warm up at least 15 minutes.

3. Stretch manifold block to first or second notches and lock pump rollers on the platen. Pump triple distilled water through the system for 10 to 15 minutes.

4. Insert reagent lines into proper reagents.

5. After about 5 minutes, turn recorder chart drive on with lower toggle switch. Adjust the recorder pen to 1 per cent transmission, with black dial on the colorimeter and "zero" blank in place.

6. Remove "zero" blank from colorimeter and by means of vernier dial set reagent base line at 97 to 99 per cent transmission. Additional electronic range expansion × 2 provides optimal sensitivity.

7. Place standards and samples on platter. Situate platter on the Sampler II with first standard or sample opposite sampling probe. Keep platter covered during sampling. Specimens are run at 30/hr. using a modified cam by cutting off every other "ear" of a 60/hr. cam. In this way the specimen is sampled for about 40 seconds and is followed by a wash of 80 seconds before the next sample is aspirated.

8. When the last sample has been recorded, turn off the chart drive and replace the "zero" blank in the colorimeter. Place all the reagent lines in

distilled water. Wash the system for at least 10 minutes or until all reagents have been washed from the system.

9. Release rollers and manifold block.

Results and Calculations

The results are read directly from the chart recordings.

IRON-BINDING CAPACITY METHOD

Principles

The Irosorb-59* test is a quick, easy, and accurate means of measuring unsaturated iron-binding capacity of the serum. The test employs radioactive iron (^{59}Fe) along with a polyether foam sponge in which is embedded a finely divided ion exchange resin, Amberlite IRA-400 type. It is a chloride form of a strongly basic anion exchange resin.

A known quantity of ^{59}Fe-labeled ferric ammonium citrate is added to serum. The iron-binding protein reacts rapidly with the ferric ion, and the iron-binding capacity is saturated by the addition of this ferric salt. The excess iron not bound to iron-binding protein is removed from the serum with the resin-sponge which absorbs the excess iron. Determination of the radioactivity remaining on the sponge allows a calculation of the absolute amount of iron which has been bound by 1 ml. of serum. This quantity is the unsaturated or latent iron-binding capacity of the serum (LIBC).

Measurement of Iron-Binding Capacity

Remove the plastic stopper (containing the resin-sponge) from a plastic tube supplied with the kit. This tube contains ^{59}Fe buffered solution. Using precision pipetting, transfer exactly 1 ml. of the patient's serum (previously warmed to room temperature) into the plastic tube and record the time. Swirl the tube to insure uniform mixing and incubate for 10 minutes. A pooled normal serum or a reference serum should also be run as a control.

Add the resin-sponge and, using the solid plastic rod supplied in the kit, push the resin-sponge down into the liquid. Expel the air from the resin-sponge by compressing it five times with the plunger. Carefully remove the plunger allowing as much serum as possible to drain back into the plastic tube. Record the time and incubate the tube for 60 minutes. Wash the plunger with iron-free water and shake off any excess water before using the plunger in the next tube.

During the hour of incubation, count the radioactivity of the tube in a suitable well-type scintillation counter for a time sufficient to obtain the desired statistical counting accuracy. One minute or 10,000 counts should be satisfactory. Obtain a background count and correct the sample count.

After the hour of incubation, wash the sponge with distilled water. Using a suitable vacuum source and a bottle trap, first aspirate the liquid from the

---

*Abbott Radiopharmaceuticals. North Chicago, Illinois.

tube and resin-sponge by means of the aspirator tip provided in the kit. Then, add 2 or 3 ml. of distilled or deionized water to the tube. Compress the resin-sponge two or three times with the plunger and aspirate the wash water. The resin-sponge should be washed and aspirated a total of three times.

Count the radioactivity remaining in the resin-sponge to the same accuracy as above and correct for background.

Calculations

Express the serum uptake as unsaturated or latent iron-binding capacity:

$$\frac{(\text{corrected original cpm}) \ \text{minus} \ (\text{corrected sponge cpm})}{\text{Corrected original cpm}} \times \text{micrograms Fe added} \times 100 = \text{micrograms LIBC/100 ml.}$$

The "micrograms Fe added" can be read from the package label.

LITHIUM

Principle

When lithium is burned in a flame its molecules are energized and emit a magenta color with a 671 mμ emission line. The intensity of this red light is proportional to the concentration of lithium in the solution being burned. Lithium in aqueous solution can be determined with negligible interference error if the following elements are present in concentrations no greater than:

1. Sodium in concentrations up to 200 times that of the lithium.
2. Calcium in concentrations up to 20 times that of the lithium.
3. Potassium in concentrations up to 5 times that of the lithium.
4. Magnesium in concentrations up to 40 times that of the lithium.

Preparation of Reagents

1. *Standard Reagent E (14.41 mEq./L. Lithium)*

    Lithium chloride (ACS Grade)   0.611 Gm.
    Distilled water, q.s.   1000.000 ml.

    Dissolve lithium chloride in distilled water and quantitatively transfer to a 1 L. volumetric flask. Dilute to volume and mix well. *Store only in Pyrex or polyethylene bottles.*

2. *Reagent 1 (1 Per Cent Sterox SE Solution)*

    Sterox SE   5 Gm.
    Distilled water, q.s.   500 ml.

    Weigh the Sterox SE into a preweighed 250 ml. beaker. Add 200 ml. of distilled water and stir to put Sterox SE into solution. Transfer quantitatively into a 500 ml. volumetric flask. Fill to the mark with distilled water and mix well.
    Store only in Pyrex or polyethylene bottles.
    NOTE: Always pour Sterox SE and distilled water *down the side of*

the neck of the flask in this and other dilutions of Sterox to prevent excessive foaming. Foaming is further minimized by filling flask nearly full before adding Sterox.

3. *Reagent 5 (0.02 Per Cent Sterox SE)*

Reagent 1 (see note under Reagent 1)	10 ml.
Distilled water, q.s.	500 ml.

Dilute reagent 1 to final volume of 500 ml. and mix well. *Store only in Pyrex or polyethylene bottles.*

4. *Reagent 19 (1.44 mEq./L. Lithium in 0.02 Per Cent Sterox SE)*

Standard reagent E	10 ml.
Reagent 1 (see note under Reagent 1)	2 ml.
Distilled water, q.s.	100 ml.

Pipet accurately the standard reagent E into a 100 ml. volumetric flask. Add reagent 1 and dilute to volume with distilled water. *Mix well and store only in Pyrex or polyethylene bottles.*

Apparatus

The following is used in lithium determinations: Coleman Model 21 Flame Photometer.

External Indicating Source.

Coleman Model 6 Junior Spectrophotometer.

Coleman Model 22 Galv-O-Meter.

Lithium filter (Catalog No. 21-211) which isolates the 671 mμ emission line.

Coleman Cat. No. 6-403 or 14-302 Scale Panel.

Operating Notes

1. Prepare the sample in aqueous solution containing 0.02 per cent Sterox. 1:1 dilution, 1 ml. of serum and 1 ml. of Sterox.

2. With the lithium filter in the flame photometer, use reagent 19 to set the indication instrument at 100 (Black Scale).

3. Use reagent 5 to set the instrument at 0 (Black Scale).

4. Atomize the prepared sample solution and record the scale reading.

Results and Calculations

Sample Scale-Reading $\times$ 10 $\times$ 1.44 = 100 mEq./L. lithium in sample solution. The lower limit of detection using this filter is 0.00140 mEq./L. (.0097 ppm) and the maximum is 140 mEq./L.

REFERENCES

CALCIUM

1. Kingsley, G. R., and Robinett, O.: New dye method for direct photometric determination of calcium. Amer. J. Clin. Path. 27: 223–230, 1957.

2. Kingsley, G. R., and Robinett, O: Further studies on a new dye method for the direct photometric determination of calcium. Amer. J. Clin. Path. 29: 171–175, 1958.

3. Klein, B., Kaufman, J. H., and Morgenstern, S.: Determination of serum calcium by automated atomic absorption spectroscopy. Clin. Chem. 13: 388–396, 1967.

4. Manson, R.: Simultaneous autoanalysis of calcium and phosphorus. Anal. Biochem. 16: 65–69, 1966.

5. Radin, N., and Granza, A. L.: Differential spectrophotometric determination of calcium. Clin. Chem. 10:704–720, 1964.

6. Wieme, R. J., and vanRaepenbush, F. R.: Automatic determination of calcium in blood and urine using Corinth Ca. Clin. Chim. Acta. 7: 883–887, 1962.

7. Wills, M. R., and Gray, B. C.: Micro-method for the estimation of calcium by Auto-Analyzer. J. Clin. Path. 17: 687–689, 1964.

INORGANIC PHOSPHATE

1. Hurst, R. O.: The determination of nucleotide phosphorus with a stannous chloride-hydrazine sulphate reagent. Canad. J. Biochem. 42: 287–292, 1964.

2. Klein, B.: Personal communication.

3. Kraml, M.: A semi-automated determination of phospholipids. Clin. Chim. Acta. 13: 442–448, 1966.

MAGNESIUM

1. Anast, C. S.: Serum magnesium levels in the newborn. Pediatrics. 33: 969–974, 1964.

2. Breen, M., and Marshall, R. T.: An automated fluorometric method for the direct determination of magnesium in serum and urine using o,o-dihydroxyazobenzene; studies on normal and uremic subjects. J. Lab. Clin. Med. 68:701–712, 1966.

3. Buhuon, C.: Microdosage du magnesium dans divers milieux biologiques. Clin. Chem. Acta. 7: 811–817, 1962.

4. Klein, B., and Oklander, M.: The automated fluorometric determination of magnesium. 11. Procedure using 8-hydroxyquinoline-5-sulfonic acid. Clin. Chem. 13: 26–35, 1967.

5. Mays, J. E., and Keele, D. K.: Serum magnesium levels in healthy children and in various disease states. Abstract. Amer. J. Dis. Child. 102: 623–624, 1961.

IRON

1. Babson, A. L., and Kleinman, N. M.: A source of error in an AutoAnalyzer determination of serum iron. Clin. Chem. 13: 163–165, 1967.

2. Fischer, D. S., and Price, D. C.: A simple serum iron method using the new sensitive chromogen tripyridyl-s-triazine Clin. Chem. 10: 21–31, 1964.

3. Koepke, J. A.: Comparison of light magnesium carbonate and amberlite sponge absorbants in the measurement of the latent iron-binding capacity of serum. Amer. J. Clin. Path. 44: 77–81, 1965.

4. Ramsay, W. N. M.: Plasma iron. In Sobatka, H., and Stewart, C. P., Advances in Clinical Chemistry, vol. 1. New York, Academic Press, Inc., 1958, pp. 1–39.

5. Young, D. S., and Hicks, J. M.: Method for the automatic determination of serum iron. J. Clin. Path. 18: 98–102, 1965.

6. Zak, B., and Epstein, E.: Automated determination of serum iron. Clin. Chem. 11: 641–644, 1965.

LITHIUM

1. Coleman Technical Report T-174-A, "Determination of Lithium with the Coleman Flame Photometer." Maywood, Illinois, Coleman Instruments, Inc.

CHAPTER V

Plasma Proteins

Clinical Annotation

THE PLASMA PROTEINS are a circulating mixture of many individual fractions. These component fractions are synthesized from amino acids derived from the proteins of food and body stores. These characteristic fractions act both as structural and functional substances. Reserve plasma proteins or protein forming materials may be stored in the liver in an amount which is several times greater than the circulating mixture. The plasma proteins also are in equilibrium with the intercellular protein pool. The biologic half life of the individual fractions varies from one to several weeks. Degradation is accomplished by hydrolysis of the protein molecules into peptides and amino acids. The chief metabolic products of this process are urea and ammonia. Measurement of total protein concentration and of individual fractions may disclose pathologic alterations of metabolic processes or of the organs that either produce or degrade protein. Methods for measuring total protein and some individual components follow.

Collection Notes

Serum or plasma is suitable for analysis; however, plasma contains fibrinogen, which is present in concentrations of 0.2 to 0.3 Gm./100 ml. and migrates as a gamma globulin. Specimens may be stored at 4° C. for several days. Repeated freezing and thawing denatures most proteins, making them unsuitable for analysis; quick freezing to -80° C. preserves most proteins indefinitely.

Interpretation of Results

The concentrations of the individual fractions vary with age, nutrition, and method of measurement. Normal values in our laboratory for serum protein fractions on cellulose acetate support media are tabulated. For the study of the individual gamma globulins, immunoelectrophoretic methods are more specific. For most plasma proteins, the concentration increases from birth to young adulthood. For gamma globulin, however, there is a physiologic decline so that the concentration of gamma globulin at 4 months is only half the concentration at birth. The usual levels are reattained at 1 or 2 years. Interpretation of an electrophoretic pattern of the plasma proteins should be made with some knowledge of the patient's clinical condition.

TOTAL PROTEIN

Principle

The biuret reaction depends upon the formation of a purple-colored complex of copper in an alkaline solution with two or more carbamyl groups (-CO-NH-)

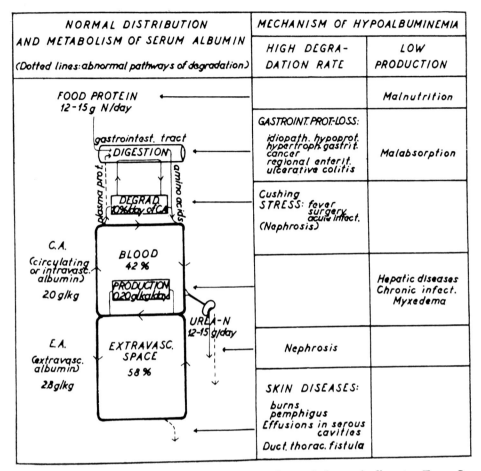

NORMAL DISTRIBUTION AND METABOLISM OF SERUM ALBUMIN (Dotted lines: abnormal pathways of degradation)	MECHANISM OF HYPOALBUMINEMIA	
	HIGH DEGRA-DATION RATE	LOW PRODUCTION
FOOD PROTEIN 12-15 g N/day		Malnutrition
gastrointest. tract →DIGESTION amino acids plasma prot. DEGRAD 10%/day of C.A.	GASTROINT. PROT.-LOSS: idiopath. hypoprot. hypertroph. gastrit. cancer regional enterit. ulcerative colitis	Malabsorption
	Cushing STRESS: fever surgery acute infect. (Nephrosis)	
C.A. (circulating or intravasc. albumin) 20 g/kg BLOOD 42 % PRODUCTION 0.20 g/kg/day URE A-N 12-15 g/day		Hepatic diseases Chronic infect. Myxedema
E.A. (extravasc. albumin) 2.8 g/kg EXTRAVASC. SPACE 58 %	Nephrosis	
	SKIN DISEASES: burns pemphigus Effusions in serous cavities Duct. thorac. fistula	

Fig. V-1. Current concept of distribution and metabolism of albumin. From S. Jarnum: Protein-Losing Gastroenteropathy. Philadelphia, F. A. Davis, 1963, p. 37.

that are joined directly together or through a single atom of nitrogen or carbon. The sample stream is diluted with an air-segmented stream of biuret reagent. The developed color is measured at 550 mμ with a flow cuvet.

Preparation of Reagents

1. *Alkaline Iodide*

Potassium iodide	10 Gm.
Sodium hydroxide	16 Gm.
Distilled water, q.s.	2000 ml.

Add 10 Gm. potassium iodide and stir until dissolved. Add 16 Gm. sodium hydroxide to approximately 800 ml. distilled water in a 1 L. volumetric flask. Stir until dissolved. Dilute to volume with distilled water, filter, and store in 1 L. polyethylene bottle.

Table V-1. Normal Adult Values of Serum Protein Fractions on Cellulose Acetate.

Protein Fraction	Percentage		Concentration (Gm./100 ml.)	
	Mean	± 2 S.D.	Mean	± 2 S.D.
Albumin	60.5%	54.3-66.7%	4.28	3.52-5.04
Alpha 1 globulin	2.8%	1.6- 4.0%	.20	.14- .28
Alpha 2 globulin	9.4%	7.0-11.8%	.66	.52- .80
Beta globulin	14.0%	11.0-17.0%	.99	.77-1.21
Gamma globulin	13.3%	8.9-17.7%	.94	.56-1.32

Table V-2. Gamma Globulin Concentrations during Infancy by Cellulose Acetate.

	Gamma Globulin (Gm./100 ml.)	
	Mean Value	Normal Range
1 week	0.7	0.4 - 0.9
1-3 mo.	0.3	0.2 - 0.4
3-6 mo.	0.4	0.2 - 0.6
6-12 mo.	0.5	0.3 - 0.7
12-18 mo.	0.6	0.4 - 0.8
18-24 mo.	0.6	0.5 - 1.1
over 2 years	Increase to normal adult values	

2. Biuret Stock Solution

Sodium potassium tartrate ($KNaC_4H_4O_6 \cdot 4H_2O$)	90 Gm.
Copper sulfate ($CuSO_4 \cdot 5H_2O$)	30 Gm.
Potassium iodide	10 Gm.
0.2 N sodium hydroxide, q.s.	2000 ml.

To 90 Gm. of sodium potassium tartrate in a 2 L. volumetric flask add 800 ml. of 0.2 N sodium hydroxide. Dissolve the tartrate and, while stirring, add 30 Gm. copper sulfate. Continue stirring until the copper sulfate is dissolved. Add 10 Gm. potasium iodide. Dissolve and dilute to 2 L. with 0.2 N sodium hydroxide. Filter and store in a polyethylene bottle.

3. Working Biuret Solution

Dilute 400 ml. of stock biuret to 2 L. with alkaline iodide solution.

4. Blank Solution

Dissolve 18 Gm. sodium potassium tartrate and dilute to 2 L. with alkaline iodide solution.

NOTE: Use this reagent in place of working biuret reagent for determining blank values on serum samples. Readjust reagent base line, determine Gm. per cent protein equivalent of blank on each specimen peak, then subtract from each biuret peak value.

5. Standards

Fifteen Gm. of carefully weighed protein is dissolved in 100 ml. of distilled water. High purity Cohn fraction V of bovine plasma is suitable. Compare this solution with College of American Pathologists total pro-

TOTAL PROTEIN

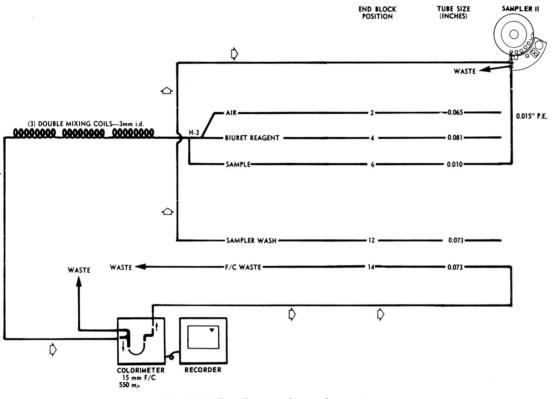

Fig. V-2. Flow diagram for total protein.

tein standards. Dilute appropriately to obtain standards of 2, 4, 6, 8, and 10 Gm./100 ml. Divide and freeze 0.2 ml. aliquots of each standard for future use.

Apparatus

The equipment used is shown in the flow diagram.

Operating Notes

1. Turn the recorder module to "on" position by moving top toggle switch upward. Do not turn chart drive on.

2. Turn colorimeter on by toggle switch opposite vernier. Let warm up at least 15 minutes.

3. Stretch manifold block to first or second notches and lock pump rollers on the platen. Pump water through system for 10 to 15 minutes.

4. Switch reagent lines to proper reagents.

5. After about 5 minutes, turn recorder chart drive on by means of lower toggle switch. Adjust the recorder pen to 1 per cent transmission with black dial on colorimeter and "zero" blank in place.

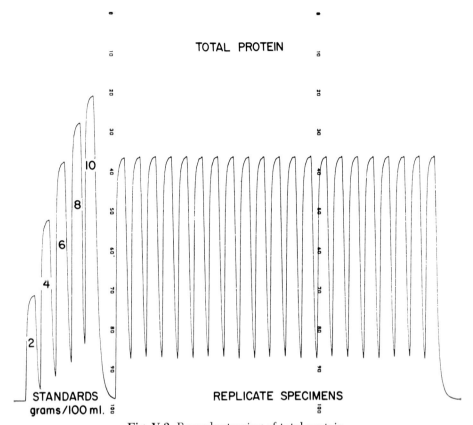

Fig. V-3. Recorder tracing of total protein.

6. Remove "zero" blank from colorimeter and by means of vernier dial set reagent base line at 97 to 99 per cent transmission.

7. Place standard and samples on platter. Situate platter on the sampler with first standard or sample opposite sampling probe. Keep platter covered during sampling.

8. Sample the specimens at the rate of 40/hr.

9. Repeat step 7, but substitute water for biuret reagent to detect those those specimens with significant "blank" values. These "blanks" are subtracted from the respective "total" protein value.

10. When last sample has been recorded, turn off the chart drive and re-place the "zero" blank in the colorimeter. Place all the reagent lines in distilled water. Wash the system for at least 10 minutes or until all reagents have been washed from the system.

11. Release rollers and manifold block.

Results and Calculations

The results are read directly from the chart recordings.

ELECTROPHORESIS OF PLASMA OR SERUM PROTEINS ON CELLULOSE ACETATE

Principle

Electrophoresis depends upon the phenomenon of charged particles in suspension or in a solution migrating in an electrical field. The direction and velocity are determined by their physical properties and by the properties of the solution. This mobility is a function of the mass, the shape, and the electrical charge of the particle, the value of the latter varying with pH. At a given pH the charge on the proteins with different isoelectric points will vary widely, but other factors may affect mobility so that different proteins migrate together and appear as a homogeneous peak in the electrophoretic pattern.

The scanning curve has a number of peaks due to the variation in color intensity of protein-dye complex bound and spread on the support medium. The number of peaks so observed corresponds to the number of electrophoretically different components present in the preparation. The area under the curve of each peak is proportional to the relative amount of each such component in the mixture.

Preparation of Reagents

1. *Barbital Buffer, pH 8.6, Ionic Strength 0.075*
   Dissolve one package of Beckman B-2 buffer in 1 L. of deionized water. The buffer must be at room temperature when used.

2. *Fixative-Dye Solution, Ponceau–S*
   The bottles supplied by Beckman are diluted to 250 ml. with distilled water. The stain contains 0.2 per cent Ponceau-S dye, 3.0 per cent trichloroacetic acid, and 3.0 per cent sulfosalicylic acid.

3. *Acetic Acid, 5 Per Cent*
   Add 50 ml. glacial acetic acid to 500 ml. of water, mix and then dilute to 1 L.

4. *Absolute Ethyl Alcohol*

5. *Clearing Solution*
   This must be made fresh daily with 25 ml. glacial acetic acid, 70 ml. ethanol, and 5 ml. distilled water.

Apparatus

A complete Beckman microzone electrophoresis cell, the Microzone Accessory Kit, and Beckman Duostat power supply are needed for electrophoretic partitioning. A Heathkit regulated power supply is an economic substitute. The Microzone Accessory Kit contains the following items:

Sample applicator, with Allen wrench; interconnecting cable for connecting Cell to Duostat; 5 stainless steel trays with covers; 2 glass drying plates; squeegee; sample covers; flat tipped tweezers; magnifying loop; wash bottle; cellulose acetate membranes; B-2 buffer; fixative-dye solution; blotters; plastic envelopes to protect finished membranes.

A recording electrophoresis densitometer is used to graph the electrophoretic pattern. We use a recording-integrating densitometer distributed by Photovolt Corp., New York (Densicord Model 542).

Operating Notes

1. *Preparation of samples and apparatus*

a. Fill electrophoresis cell with buffer, pour buffer solution through siphon tube to eliminate air bubbles. Thoroughly wipe off any which has splashed on the partition of the cell or around the siphon because the buffer will conduct current between the two reservoirs when power is applied to the cell.

b. Fill prebuffering tray with 40 ml. of B-2 buffer.

c. Fill fixative-dye solution tray with 50 ml. of dye solution. Dye may be used several times, but do not put used dye in container with fresh dye.

d. Fill acetic acid rinse tray with 50 ml. 5 per cent acetic acid.

e. Fill ethanol tray with 50 ml. ethanol.

f. Fill clearing solution tray with freshly prepared solution, and place the glass plate in the bottom of the tray.

g. Check condition of the applicator-tip; this is extremely fragile.

h. Install the membrane in the prebuffering tray by letting it float on the surface of the buffer. Use the tweezers to lower the membrane onto the buffer so that air bubbles are not trapped under the membrane. If bubbles are trapped, discard and start again with a fresh membrane. Allow membrane to become thoroughly wet and then blot between the special blotters provided for just a few seconds—just enough to remove the surface liquid.

i. Install membrane on the bridge and place it in the cell. Be sure the membrane is not touching any surface of the cell. Connect cell to power supply and allow 2 minutes for equilibration. Read instructions in manual about power supply connections.

2. *Application of Sample*

a. Arrange serum drops on nonporous (eg., Parafilm, dividing paper from membranes, etc.) paper.

b. Apply samples as quickly as possible to avoid needless evaporation and to minimize diffusion of sample in membrane before current is applied. In order, pick up sample by moving the tip slowly across the top surface of the sample drop. Place applicator across the cell in the appropriate positioning slot. Touch the button to release sample. Wait 5 seconds, retract tip, wash off tip with distilled water. Be careful not to damage tip as it is very fragile.

c. Apply the remaining seven samples in the same fashion, being careful to wash the tip between applications and to replace cell cover between applications.

3. *Electrophoresis*

a. Set the power supply for constant voltage, turn on current, and adjust to 250 volts.

b. Check starting current by changing the meter range switch to 10 to 15 mA. If the cell is operating properly, a current of 3.5 to 5.8 mA will be obtained. If not, refer to the manual instead of continuing.

c. Change the power supply back to constant voltage and continue the run for 24 minutes.

d. Stop the current by turning the output adjust control to the left until the light goes out.

e. Detach plug from the cell and proceed with staining.

4. *Staining, fixing, and clearing*

a. Remove the membrane from the bridge with tweezers and slip the membrane into the dye solution tray. Submerge completely and stain for 10 minutes. Be sure no air bubbles are trapped under the membrane.

b. Rinse membrane 3 to 4 times in 5 per cent acetic acid. Rinse until no more stain is eluted from the membrane.

c. Transfer to ethanol and agitate for 1 minute.

d. Transfer to clearing solution and agitate for 1 minute.

e. Position membrane over glass plate and lift both out of the tray. Drain off excess clearing solution and squeeze gently.

f. Air dry for 30 minutes at room temperature.

g. Carefully peel membrane off the glass plate and place in protective clear plastic cover. Do not handle the membrane, especially over the protein bands.

5. *Scanning*

a. Turn power switch to "on" position on Densicord and Integraph. Allow to "warm-up" for 20 minutes.

b. Check chart paper to insure that it is aligned properly on the sprockets with the tear-off bar secure in the two buttons on the instrument.

c. Check the phototube unit to see that the correct filter ($545 \, m\mu$) is in place.

d. Test the "tracing" and "pipping" device pens to see that they are working properly.

e. Introduce the acetate membrane to be analyzed into the frame, checking that the slit of the phototube is aligned with the proper electrophoresis strip.

f. Turn on pen and chart toggle switches.

g. Check zero adjustment of the integrator. Less than 1 pip per 20 seconds indicates a reasonable adjustment.

h. Set the "response" control to the appropriate setting. Setting number "5" is an approximation of suitable absorbance. Refer to section on "Calibration" in instrument manual. Then switch the Densicord to "integrate."

i. Turn the bottom ring of "dark point" control, if necessary, to bring the pen into 50 to 80 division range.

j. Set "damping" control approximately two-thirds clockwise and turn "vibration" control back and forth to observe that a periodic vibration (dither) is impressed on the pen. Set the control to a point in which the pen point "wiggle" is just noticeable.

k. Turn the "damping" control counterclockwise until the pen just begins to oscillate. Turn back approximately 15 degrees (clockwise) to keep the pen

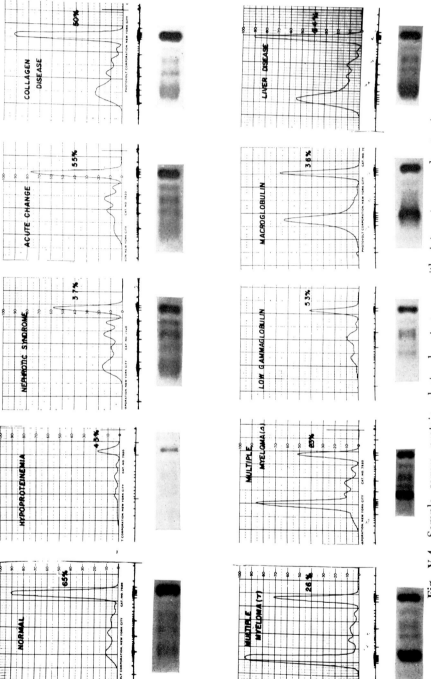

Fig. V-4. Sample serum protein electrophoretograms with integrator-recorder tracings.

action lively, yet safely below level of oscillation. Do not confuse oscillation with the small pen-dither described above.

l. Turn the exact dark point (100 division mark on scale), using both the coarse (bottom ring) and fine adjustments (upper knob) of "dark point" control.

m. Now return carriage to the starting point. For the next step, it is important to have a clear area presented to the photometer which is representative of the *background*. Therefore, place the carriage in a way that a clean area, free of color bands, rips, dirt, etc., is above the slit. It is advisable to turn off "chart" switch during the operation of this step.

n. Swing arm down and push knob in all the way. Then adjust "full light" controls (bottom, coarse; top knob, fine) until the pen is exactly on the 0 division mark at the right-hand edge of the chart. Pull out knob and readjust the dark point (other edge of the chart) if necessary. Repeat this process to make sure the Densicord is properly set for these extremes. Observe that the pen moves across the chart paper rapidly. If sluggishness is observed, decrease damping or increase pen vibration appropriately.

o. The Densicord is now ready for operation. Make sure that shutter knob is all the way *in* and the chart switch is *on*. The instrument will automatically scan and record the curves.

Results and Calculations

Electrophoretograms with integrated tracings are obtained. Divide plot into components by drawing vertical lines to integrator blips in "valleys" between all component peaks. Count and record integration "blips" between the vertical lines for each component. For percentage of each component, divide the individual number of "blips" of an area by the total number of "blips." For Gm./100 ml. of each protein electrophoretic fraction, multiply individual fraction percentages by the total protein in Gm./100 ml. After reporting results, file the membrane and identification card for future reference. Some feel that there is no good reason to quantitate the individual proteins on the electrophoretic patterns. Rather they feel an examination of the over-all pattern is of more value to the clinician. Some typical patterns are illustrated.

ELECTROPHORESIS OF SERUM LIPOPROTEINS ON PAPER

Principle

Electrophoretic fractionation of the serum lipoproteins is performed on paper, as are serum proteins. The individual lipids are developed by a lipophilic stain. The color intensity of the separate lipid bands is proportional to their separate concentrations.

Preparation of Reagents

1. *Sodium barbital buffer, pH 8.6 0.075 ionic strength:*

Diethyl barbitaric acid	2.76 Gm.
Sodium diethylbarbiturate	15.40 Gm.

Distilled water, q.s.   1000.00 ml.

Dissolve the dry ingredients in distilled water and dilute to 1 L.

2. *Fat Red 7B Stain*

A stock solution of stain is prepared by saturating absolute ethyl alcohol with fat red 7B (Ciba). Subsequently, a working stain is made by adjusting the alcohol to a 60 per cent solution with water; then, the excess dye is removed by double filtration (Whatman #1).

Apparatus

Spinco Model R paper electrophoresis cell, power supply and accessories are used. A ventilated drying oven at 120 to 130° C. is used for drying and fixing the protein on the paper supports.

Operating Notes

1. Allow barbital buffer to thoroughly wet the Schleicher and Schuell support papers.

2. Allow equilibration and uniform saturation of papers by maintaining constant current at 2.5 m.a.

3. Discontinue current and apply 30 μL. serum in 10 μL. aliquots to center of strip with the sample applicator.

4. Maintain a constant current of 2.5 m.a. for 17 to 18 hr.

5. Discontinue current, place electrophoretic strips on drying rack, and place in preheated oven at 120 to 130° C.

6. When strips are dry, stain as follows:

a. Immerse in working dye solution at room temperature for 1 hr.

b. Transfer to decolorizing bath consisting of a 0.1 per cent solution of 5 per cent sodium hypochloride in a 2 per cent acetic acid solution for 1 to 2 minutes.

c. Before the background is completely decolorized, transfer to a 2 per cent acetic acid solution and rinse thoroughly for 1 to 2 minutes.

d. This bath is followed by three additional 15-minute rinses (45 minutes) of fresh 2 per cent acetic acid. Agitate occasionally.

e. Air dry strips in horizontal position.

7. The individual paper electrophoretic strips are scanned in a recording densitometer (Analytrol RB) using two 500 mμ interference filters and a B-2 cam.

Results and Calculations

There is no ideal standard for this form of lipoprotein analysis. However, in order to establish a point of reference, a pseudostandard is used. Pream®, a readily obtained dried cream, is highly stainable; 0.3 Gm. diluted in 20 ml. of water is a satisfactory monitor or standard.

FIBRINOGEN

Clinical Annotation and Interpretation of Results

Fibrinogen in concentrations between 150 and 350 mg./100 ml. is present in the plasma of normal individuals. In acquired coagulation disorders (e.g., defibrination syndrome), and in congenital hypofibrinogenemia, it is present in lesser amounts. Typically increased levels are seen in pregnancy. This method yields somewhat lower levels than several other fibrinogen procedures, but it has the advantage of simplicity and speed of performance.

Principle

Fibrinogen is precipitated from plasma as a suspension of fine particles by the action of a special reagent. The resulting turbidity is estimated spectrometrically.

Preparation of Reagents

1. *Parfentjev's Reagent*

Ammonium sulfate	133.330 Gm.
Sodium chloride	10.110 Gm.
Merthiolate	0.025 Gm.
Distilled water, q.s.	1000.000 ml.

Dissolve dry reagents in water and dilute to volume of 1 L.

2. *Fibrinogen (Warner-Chilcott)*

Dilute the lyophilized fibrinogen very gently, and prepare a 300 mg. per cent standard as well as 150 mg. and 75 mg. standards by serial dilution.

Apparatus

A Coleman Jr. (Model 6A) spectrophotometer is used to read optical density.

Specimen Collection

4.5 ml. of blood is anticoagulated with 0.5 ml. of 4 per cent sodium citrate. This is easily accomplished using a prothrombin Vacutainer®.

Operating Notes

1. The supernatant plasma is obtained by centrifugation at 2500 rpm for 10 minutes.

2. The blank and samples are set up as follows:

Blank: 0.5 ml. plasma + 4.5 ml. normal saline
Sample: 0.5 ml. plasma + 4.5 ml. of ammonium sulfate reagent
Normal control: 0.5 ml. plasma + 4.5 ml. of ammonium sulfate reagent

3. The spectrophotometer is set at 100 per cent transmittance at a wavelength of 510 mμ with the blank.

4. The optical density of the sample is read exactly 3 minutes after its

formation. If the sample has clotted prior to reading, the sample is given a vigorous shake just before the reading is taken.

5. Construct a standard curve using the same procedure as described for the samples.

Results and Calculations

The fibrinogen concentration is determined by reading the optical density of the unknown against the standard curve.

MEASUREMENT OF GASTROINTESTINAL PROTEIN LOSS IN INTESTINAL DISORDERS

(Use of ^{51}Cr-Albumin in Exudative Enteropathy)

Principle

Significant gastrointestinal loss of protein has been shown to occur in a variety of clinical disorders; this phenomena is now called exudative enteropathy. That this process could occur and cause hypoproteinemia is not surprising since the surface area of the intestine is approximately five times that of the skin. The rapid digestion of proteins by the enzymes normally present in the gastrointestinal tract requires the use of an indirect method to measure this loss. ^{51}Cr-albumin is injected into the plasma protein pool, and its loss into the gut is measured quantitatively by the recovery of ^{51}Cr label in the stool. This is facilitated by the fact that chromium forms insoluble salts in the intestine that are not reabsorbed. ^{51}Cr-albumin supersedes the older and less satisfactory agents (eg., ^{131}I -PVP, ^{131}I -albumin, immunologic methods, etc.).

Procedure

1. Apply a urine-collection device to males or an indwelling Foley catheter to females.

2. Administer 0.5 μc. ^{51}Cr-albumin per Kg. body weight intravenously by rapid injection, but limit maximum dose to 20 μc. Dilute dose with isotonic saline so that at least 2 ml. is administered; use plastic syringe to diminish loss of tracer by glass absorption. At the same time set aside an identical amount of the dose in a 2 L. plastic bottle to be used as standard.

3. Save all urine and stools separately for 72 hr.; it is essential that the urine does not contaminate the stool. Pool stool collections in a 2 L. plastic bottle, the entire top cut off to facilitate collections. Seal with tape between additions. Infant stool collections are facilitated by use of paper diapers and cutting away the unsoiled portions. Pool urine specimens; no preservatives are required.

Interpretation of Results

	% Dose in 72 hr. Urine	% Dose in 72 hr. Stool
Normal	10-15	less than 1
Exudative Enteropathy	6-12	2 - 20

REFERENCES

TOTAL PROTEIN

1. Mabry, C. C., Gevedon, R. E., Roeckel, I. E., and Gochman, N.: Automated submicro-chemistries: A system of rapid submicrochemical analysis for the measurement of sodium, potassium, chloride, carbon dioxide, sugar, urea nitrogen, total and direct-reacting bilirubin and total protein. Amer. J. Clin. Path. 46:265–281, 1966.

PROTEIN ELECTROPHORESIS

1. Briere, R. O., and Mull, J. D.: Electrophoresis of serum protein with cellulose acetate. A method for quantitation. Amer. J. Clin. Path. 42: 547–551, 1964.

2. Dirstine, P. H., MacCallum, D. B., Anson, J. H., and Mohammed, A.: Optimum clinical applications of serum protein in electrophoresis. Clin. Chem. 10: 853–861, 1964.

3. Grunbaum, B. W., Lyons, M. F., Carroll, N. V., and Zec, J.: Quantitative analysis of normal human serum proteins on permanently transparentized cellulose acetate membranes. Microchim. J. 7:54–56, 1963.

4. Kohn, J.: Cellulose acetate electrophoresis and immuno diffusion techniques. *In* Chromatographic and Electrophoretic Techniques, ed. I, Smith Edition II. New York, Interscience Publishers, Inc., 1960, pp. 56.

5. Korotzer, J. L., Bergquist, L. M., and Searcy, R. L.: Use of cellulose acetate and Ponceau S for electrophoretic serum protein analysis. Amer. J. Med. Techn. 27: 197–203, 1961.

6. Ritts, Jr., R. E., and Ondrick, F. W.: Electrophoresis of serum proteins on cellulose acetate. Techn. Bull. Regist. Med. Techn. 34: 21–31, 1964.

7. Sheperd, H. G., and Mason, C. C.: Normal electrophoretic values of human serum proteins eluted from cellulose acetate membranes. Amer. J. Clin Pat. 43:464–466, 1965.

8. Sunderman, F. W., Jr.: Studies of the serum proteins. VI. Recent advances in clinical interpretation of electrophoretic fractionations. Amer. J. Clin. Path. 42: 1–21, 1964.

9. Sunderman, Jr., F. W., Sunderman, F. W.: Clinical applications of the fractionation of serum proteins by paper electrophoresis. Amer. J. Clin. Path. 27: 125–158, 1957.

10. Sunderman, Jr., F. W., Sunderman, F. W.: Studies of the serum proteins IV. The dye binding of purified serum proteins separated by continuous-flow electrophoresis. Clin. Chem. 5: 171–185, 1959.

LIPOPROTEIN ELECTROPHORESIS

1. Straus, R., and Wurm, M.: A new staining procedure and a method for quantitation of serum lipoproteins separated by paper electrophoresis. Amer. J. Clin. Path. 29:581–589, 1958.

FIBRINOGEN

1. Fowell, A. H.: Turbidimetric method of fibrinogen assay. Amer. J. Clni. Path. 25: 340–342, 1955.

[51]CHROMIUM-ALBUMIN FOR GI PROTEIN LOSS

1. Mabry, C. C., Greenlaw, R. H., and DeVore, W. D.: Measurement of gastrointestinal loss of plasma albumin; a clinical and laboratory evaluation of [51]chromium-labeled albumin. J. Nucl. Med. 6: 93–108, 1965.

2. Rubini, M. E., and Sheehy, T. W.: Exudative enteropathy. I. A comparative study of Cr[51]-Cl and I[131] PVP. J. Lab. Clin. Med. 58:892–901, 1961.

3. Waldman, T. A.: Gastrointestinal protein-loss demonstrated by Cr[51]-labeled albumin. Lancet. 2: 121–123, 1961.

CHAPTER VI

Enzymes

Clinical Annotation

MANY ENZYMES are normally present and measurable in plasma or serum. They arise from the normal breakdown and turnover of tissues, and their concentrations in plasma are greatly less than their intracellular concentrations. The elevations of plasma enzymes in the course of disease are usually the result of tissue insult with leakage of enzymes out of the damaged cells. The elevation of alkaline phosphatase in rickets, however, is associated with an increase in the activity of osteoblasts. These cells are rich in alkaline phosphatase, and excess plasma alkaline phosphatase is derived from local overproduction of the enzyme by highly active or increased numbers of osteoblasts. Although enzymes are present in all tissues, specific enzymes are uniquely rich in certain tissues and organs. Thus, elevations of these enzymes in serum are characteristic of injury to that tissue or organ. This phenomenon accounts for the diagnostic value of serum enzyme measurements.

The same serum enzyme activity may arise from different tissues, but, on occasion, an enzyme from one tissue can be chemically distinguished from another although they catalyze the same reaction. Their different characteristics may be elucidated by their activity in the presence of inhibitors or varying substrates. Importantly, there may be multiple forms, isozymes. They differ from each other in certain properties and tissues of greatest concentration, although they catalyze the same reaction. The enzyme measurements described in the subsequent pages represent only a small proportion of enzymes available for use in diagnosis and management, but they are a representative "battery" with which there is considerable clinical correlation and experience.

Collection Notes

When blood is collected, care must be taken to avoid hemolysis. Erythrocytes themselves are rich in certain enzymes such as acid phosphatase, the transaminases, cholinesterase and aldolase; their rupture will cause factitial increases in concentrations in serum. On the other hand, moderate hemolysis does not affect such serum enzymes as alkaline phosphatase and creatine phosphokinase. Although serum is generally preferred, plasma can be used for enzyme assays. If plasma is used, the choice of an anticoagulant is important (e.g., oxalate inhibits LDH activity; oxalate, citrate, and heparin do not affect GOT or GPT activity).

Interpretation of Results

Enzymes are quantitated by their enzymatic activity; namely, as the quantity of substrate which is converted to the end product by the enzyme in a given

Table VI-1.—Relation of Conventional Enzyme Units to International Units

Enzyme	Conventional Units (method by which unit expresses enzyme activity)	Equivalent in I.U. (μM/min/L)
Alkaline phosphatase	King-Armstrong unit (1 mg. phenol/15 min./100 ml. with phenylphosphate as substrate)	7.2
	Bodansky unit (1 mg. phosphate P/hr./100 ml. with β-glycerophosphate as substrate)	5.35
	Bessey-Lowry-Brock unit (mMole p-nitrophenol/hr./100 ml. with p-nitro phenylphosphate as substrate)	16.7
Acid phosphatase	King-Armstrong unit (1 mg. phenol/hr./100 ml. with phenylphosphate as substrate)	1.8
	Bodansky unit (1 mg. phosphate P/hr./100 ml. with β glycerophosphate as substrate)	5.35
Transaminases (GPT and GOT)	Spectrophotometric unit (change of 0.001 in optical density at 340 mμ/min./ml.)	0.48
Lactate dehydrogenase	Spectrophotometric unit (change of 0.001 in optical density at 340 mμ/min./ml.)	0.48
Aldolase	Sibley and Lehninger unit (Warburg Technique) (splitting of 1 μl fructose 1:6 diphosphate sol./hr./ml.)	0.74
	Schapira unit (1 mg. triose phosphate P/min./ml.)	16.0
	Bruns unit (splitting of 0.44 μ moles of fructose 1:6 diphosphate/hr./ml.)	0.74
Amylase	Somogyi unit (that activity which digests 5 mg. starch/15 min./100 ml.)	20.6

(From Howell, J. Pediat. 68:121, 1966.)

time under standard conditions. Thus, we are always indicating enzyme activity, not absolute quantities of enzyme. The units in which enzyme activity is expressed vary widely and depend primarily on the investigators who first worked with the enzyme. Thus, it is difficult to compare accurately the units obtained with different methods. Recently it has been advocated that enzyme activities be expressed in "international units." An international unit (I.U.) equals 1 μmole of substrate transformed or of product formed per minute. Units can be expressed per milliliter or per liter.

In view of the wide variety of methods available, it is essential to know the normal range of values for the methods used in each laboratory. Ranges of normal values for serum enzyme measurements performed in our laboratory with the methods to be described are presented with explanation in the subsequent addendum.

Clinical Annotation Addendum

1. *Alkaline phosphatase*. Though the specific function of alkaline phosphatase in bone formation is unknown, the association of alkaline phosphatase with osteoblasts and chondrocytes during bone formation under all conditions is well established. The rapid rate of bone growth in children is reflected in the fact that serum alkaline phosphatase is higher in children than in adults. If growth is interrupted as in hypothroidism or cystic fibrosis, serum alkaline phosphatase falls to normal adult levels. Serum alkaline phosphatase is greatly elevated in vitamin-D-deficiency rickets and Paget's disease. Elevated levels are also seen in hyperparathyroidism, healing fractures, certain tumors which have metastasized to bone, and disorders of the hepatobiliary system. Very low levels are observed in scurvy and negligible levels in congenital hypophosphatasia. Normal values in our laboratory are listed in tabular form as Bessey-Lowry-Brock units:

Micro Automated Serum (Plasma) Alkaline Phosphatase Assay			
	# Normal Tested	Mean	SD	Range
Prematures (birth to 6 wk.)	12	11.1	3.8	5.2–16.5
Term newborns (1 day to 1 mo.)	14	7.7	2.5	3.0–13.0
Infants (1 mo. to 2 yr.)	17	12.3	4.1	5.7–19.6
Young children (2 yr. to 10 yr.)	14	10.1	3.3	5.9–13.9
Older children (10 yr. to 18 yr.)	12	8.4	2.9	5.6–14.0
Young adults (18 yr. to 45 yr.)	23	3.5	0.9	1.2– 5.1
Older adults (45 yr. and older)	13	3.8	1.0	2.3– 5.2

For comparison of these alkaline phosphatase values with values obtained by other methods, the following experience is shown:

	Values on Same Sera	
	Serum No. 1	Serum No. 2
Bodansky unit	2.6	14.0
King-Armstrong unit	5.7	20.5
Bessey-Lowry-Brock unit (A-M-P buffer)	3.1	18.2

A rule of thumb conversion ratio is 0.8 Bod. units = 1.7 KA units = 1 BLB unit.

2. *Glutamic oxaloacetic transaminase (GOT) and glutamic pyruvate transaminase (GPT)*. These enzymes are of particular value in the diagnosis of liver disease. The heart and kidney are relatively rich sources of GOT, but the liver is the principal source of GPT. In acute liver cell injury, as occurs in hepatitis, changes in GOT and GPT levels closely parallel each other, but the rise in GOT usually exceeds that of GPT. Though GOT is elevated in myocardial and skeletal muscle diseases, more specific enzymes for those tissues are more useful. GOT in the blood of newly born infants is above adult levels, but progressively declines to adult levels at about 3 months of age. Normal values as measured in our laboratory are:

Glutamic Oxaloacetic Transaminase (GOT)	
Newborn to 3 mo.	5–120 spectrophotometric or fluorometric units/ml. (Karmen)
3 mo. to adult	5–40 spectrophotometric or fluorometric units/ml. (Karmen)

Glutamic Pyruvate Transaminase (GPT)	
Newborn to 3 mo.	5–90 spectrophotometric or fluorometric units/ml. (Wroblewski)
3 mo. to adult	5–40 spectrophotometric or fluorometric units/ml. (Wroblewski)

3. *Lactate dehydrogenase (LDH)*. LDH elevation is relatively nonspecific and occurs in a wide variety of diseases. It is especially useful in hemolytic anemia as elevated values are commonly found. Such levels also occur in certain cases of widely disseminated malignant disease. Moderately elevated values occur after myocardial infarction; the test is of particular value in this context since the elevation persists up to ten days or more after the acute episode. In liver diseases, elevated values may be found in about 70 per cent of cases of acute hepatitis, infectious mononucleosis, and other acute infections; normal values usually occur in obstructive jaundice, compensated cirrhosis, and chronic infective conditions.

LDH consists of five isoenzymes separable by electrophoresis and other means. The electrophoretically slowest fraction, LDH_5, is abundant in liver and skeletal muscle, while that found in the heart and erythrocytes consists mostly of LDH_1. LDH_1 is more stable than LDH_5. The serum LDH in acute liver disease is thus more sensitive to heat inhibition than that in myocardial infarction.

Normal values in the newly born and young individual are greater than in older persons. Suitable "total" LDH normal levels are:

Lactate Acid Dehydrogenase (LDH)	
Newborn	440–2540 spectrophotometric or fluorometric units
0 to 30 days	240–1021 spectrophotometric or fluorometric units
1 mo. to 2 yr.	200– 640 spectrophotometric or fluorometric units
2 yr. to 12 yr.	110– 500 spectrophotometric or fluorometric units
12 yr. to adult	50– 250 spectrophotometric or fluorometric units

4. *Amylase*. α-Amylase, an enzyme which hydrolyzes polysaccharides as glycogen, starches, etc., has its greatest concentrations in the pancreas and salivary glands. Sudden, greatly elevated levels occur in acute pancreatitis. At the onset of mumps serum amylase is usually elevated, but by the end of the second week the serum level returns to normal. Morphine and codeine, by closing the sphincter of Oddi, increase the intraductal pressure in the pancreas and can cause significant elevations of plasma amylase. These increases in plasma amylase are usually maximal five hours after administration of the drug and return to normal within twenty-four hours. Corticosteroids increase serum levels of amylase, while infusion of carbohydrates lowers the serum levels. Amylase is not detectable in the serum of newborn infants; it first appears at

about 2 months. By one year of age the serum level compares with that of the normal adult. Normal values are:

	Amylase	
Birth to 1 yr.	0–127	Somogyi units
1 yr. to 12 yr.	8–183	Somogyi units
12 yr. to adult	19–103	Somogyi units

5. *Aldolase*. This enzyme has proved to be of value in the differential diagnosis of muscular disease. It is abundant in muscle, although lesser amounts are widely distributed in other tissues. As erythrocytes contain considerable aldolase, hemolysis must be carefully avoided in serum used for this assay. Aldolase activity in serum declines from birth to adolescence, and, in the first two years of life, normal female serum values are 15 to 35 per cent higher than those of the male.

Progressive muscular dystrophy in its active stages regularly produces greatly elevated serum levels of aldolase. These enzyme levels gradually decline and reach low levels in bedridden patients. Serum aldolase is elevated in hepatitis, but is not as useful in the diagnosis of liver disease as are the transaminases. Liver aldolase is much less active than muscle aldolase when fructose-1:6-diphosphate is used as substrate rather than fructose-1-phosphate. Normal values are:

	Aldolase
0 to 2 yr.	2–25 Sibley-Lehninger units/ml.
2 to 5 yr.	3–18 Sibley-Lehninger units/ml.
5 to 15 yr.	4–17 Sibley-Lehninger units/ml.
Adult	3–15 Sibley-Lehninger units/ml.

6. *Creatine phosphokinase (CPK)*. The highest concentrations of this enzyme occur in striated muscle, although lesser amounts are present in the heart and cerebral cortex. The absence of CPK in liver and erythrocytes avoids any confusion which might arise through liver disease or hemolysis. CPK is greatly elevated in progressive muscular dystrophy as is aldolase. In patients with neurogenic muscular atrophy, there are no or only negligible elevations of serum CPK levels. CPK can be moderately elevated immediately following strenuous muscular activity; thus, exericse must be avoided prior to obtaining samples. Normal values are:

Creatine Phosphokinase (CPK)	
Newborn	1–12 I.U.
Infant to adult	
female	< 2 I.U.
male	< 3 I.U.

7. *Acid phosphatase*. Elevation of serum acid phosphatase, which is inhibited by adding L-tartrate, is regularly seen in metastatic carcinoma of the pancreas. In Gaucher's disease, serum acid phosphatase is moderately elevated and, it is not tartrate labile. This increase in serum acid phosphatase can be demon-

strated only when phenylphosphate is used as substrate. High levels of acid phosphatase have been found in osteopetrosis and in some children with osteogenesis imperfecta. The total acid phosphatase activity is high in the sera of newborn infants, declines slightly during the first two weeks, and then declines gradually to adult levels in late adolescence.

Acid Phosphatase	
Newborn to 2 wk.	2–9 King-Armstrong Units
2 wk. to 18 yr.	2–7 King-Armstrong Units
Adult	1–3 King-Armstrong Units

ALKALINE PHOSPHATASE

Principle

Alkaline phosphatase acts at pH 10.25 to liberate (by hydrolysis) p-nitro-phenol from disodium p-nitrophenylphosphate. The p-nitrophenol released is measured spectrometrically to determine alkaline phosphatase activity.

Preparation of Reagents

1. *50 per cent Amino-Methyl-Propanol (W/V)*

2-amino-2-methyl-1-propanol	500 Gm.
Distilled water, q.s.	1000 ml.

Melt the amino-methyl-propanol and weigh. Transfer to a 1000 ml. volumetric flask and add distilled water. Mix, dilute to volume, and label properly.

2. *Buffer 0.05 M (pH 10.25)*

Stock amino-methyl-propanol, 50 per cent	190 ml.
Hydrochloric acid, 5 N	approx. 22 ml.
Distilled water, q.s.	2000 ml.

Transfer amino-methyl-propanol to a 2 L. volumetric flask. Add approximately 600 ml. of water. Mix thoroughly. Add 5 N HCl until the pH is brought to 10.25. Usually 22 to 26 ml. is required. Dilute to volume with water and mix thoroughly. This solution *must* be kept under refrigeration; it is stable under these conditions for about six months.

3. *Buffered Substrate*

Disodium p-nitrophenylphosphate	1.0 Gm.
Magnesium chloride, 1 M	0.5 ml.
Buffer, pH 10.25, q.s.	500.0 ml.

Place approximately 450 ml. of buffer (pH 10.25) in a 500 ml. volumetric flask. Add exactly 1 Gm. of disodium p-nitrophenyl-phosphate (weighed on an analytical balance) and mix well. Add 0.5 ml. of magnesium chloride and dilute to volume with buffer (pH 10.25). This reagent is stable for three days if returned to the refrigerator (5° C.) after use.

4. *Magnesium Chloride Solution, 1 M*

Magnesium chloride	9.52 Gm.
Hydrochloric acid, conc.	2.00 drops
Distilled water, q.s.	100.00 ml.

Dry the magnesium chloride in an oven at 110° C. overnight. Dissolve the weighed magnesium chloride in about 80 ml. of distilled water in a 100 ml. volumetric flask. Add the concentrated HCl and dilute to volume with water. Mix thoroughly.

5. *Stock Standard (10 mM/L.)*

p-nitrophenol	139.1 mg.
Buffer (pH 10.25) q.s.	100.0 ml.

Dissolve the p-nitrophenol in buffer in a 100 ml. volumetric flask and dilute to volume. This stock solution must be refrigerated.

6. *Working Standards*

Working standards are as follows:

Stock Solution Added (ml.)	Dilute with Buffer to (ml.)	p-nitrophenol Value (mM/L.)
0.25	10.0	0,25
0.5	10.0	0.5
1.0	10.0	1.0
1.5	10.0	1.5
2.0	10.0	2.0
2.5	10.0	2.5
3.0	10.0	3.0
4.0	10.0	4.0

NOTE: Incubation time must be taken into account as the BLB unit is expressed as substrate liberated in 1 hr.; more precisely, one BLB unit equals 1 mM/L. of p-nitrophenol liberated at 37° C. in 1 hr. Therefore the final result will entail calculating the value in terms of one hour's incubation. These calculations must be incorporated into the p-nitrophenol standards in order for the technologist to be able to read the results directly without applying the correction factor. Thus, if the time in the dialyzer and 37° C. waterbath is 14.3 minutes, the incubation factor is 60/14.3 minutes or 4.2. These adjusted values are used on each of the p-nitrophenol working standards as well as their value in terms of enzyme activity using our present manifold. This eliminates applying a factor to the unknowns.

Actual Value of p-nitrophenol present	Value in Terms of Enzyme Activity
mM/L.	mM/L.
0.25 × 4.2 =	1.05
0.5	2.1
1.0	4.2
1.5	6.3
2.0	8.4
2.5	10.5
3.0	12.6
4.0	16.8

ALKALINE PHOSPHATASE

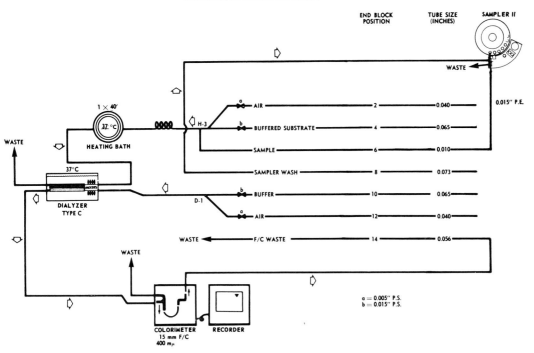

Fig. VI-1.—Flow diagram for alkaline phosphatase.

Apparatus

A basic unit is employed for the alkaline phosphatase plus heating bath for the incubation.

Operating Notes

1. Turn the recorder module to "on" position by moving top toggle switch upward. Do not turn chart drive on.

2. Turn colorimeter on by toggle switch opposite vernier. Let warm up at least 15 minutes.

3. Stretch manifold block to first or second notches and lock pump rollers on the platen. Pump water through system for 10 to 15 minutes.

4. Switch reagent lines to proper reagents.

5. After about 5 minutes, turn recorder chart drive on by means of lower toggle switch. Adjust the recorder pen to 99 per cent transmission or 0.01 O.D. with black dial on colorimeter.

6. Remove "zero" blank from colorimeter and by means of vernier dial set reagent baseline to desired setting.

7. Place standards and samples on platter. Situate platter on the sampler with first standard or sample opposite sampling probe. Keep platter covered during sampling.

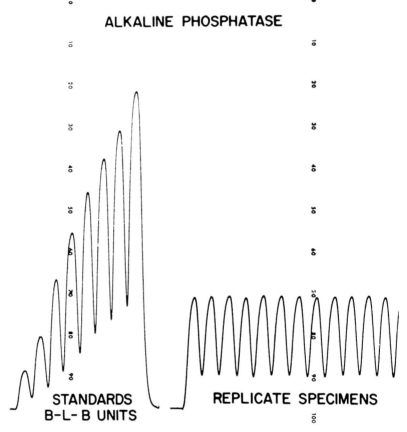

Fig. VI-2.—Recorder tracing for alkaline phosphatase.

8. Sample the specimens at the rate of 40/hr.

9. When last sample has been recorded, turn off the chart drive and replace the "zero" blank in the colorimeter. Place all the reagent lines in distilled water. Wash the system for at least 20 minutes or until all reagents have been washed from the system.

10. Release rollers and manifold block.

11. The colorimeter is fitted with 400 mμ interference filters.

12. An in-serum standard or control *must* be included in each run. These enzyme controls are necessary because p-nitrophenol standards are not derived from serum or plasma. The standards could appear normal even though specimen samples were inhibited by improper collection techniques, etc.

Calculations and Results

The unknown values are read directly from the recorder chart.

LACTATE DEHYDROGENASE (LDH)

Principle

$$\underset{\text{Lactate}}{CH_3 \cdot CHOH \cdot COO^-} + NAD \overset{LDH}{\rightleftharpoons} \underset{\text{Pyruvate}}{CH_3CO \cdot COO^-} + NADH_2$$

Lactate dehydrogenase (LDH) activity may be determined in either of two ways, according to the direction of the reaction. Lactate or pyruvate may be used as substrate with NAD or $NADH_2$ as coenzyme respectively; however, optimum conditions are quite different for the two reactions. The method described is by the forward lactate → pyruvate reaction. Enzyme activity is determined by measuring the fluorescence of $NADH_2$ formed after a fixed incubation time. $NADH_2$ is fluorescent (peak at about 470 mμ) when excited by light at 340 mμ, whereas NAD is not.

Preparation of Reagents

1. *0.05 M Tris Buffer (pH 7.6)*

Tris (Hydroxy-methyl) amino-methane	12.1 Gm.
Distilled water, q.s.	2000.0 ml.

Dissolve tris (hydroxy-methyl) amino methane in approximately 1800 ml. of distilled water. Adjust pH to 7.6 with conc. HCl, then dilute with water to final volume of 2 L.

2. *0.075 M L-lactate in 0.05 M Tris Buffer (pH 7.6)*

Tris (Hydroxy-methyl) amino-methane	6.05	Gm.
Lactic acid, 85 per cent	15.90	ml.
Hydroxylamine hydrochloride	0.695	Gm.
Distilled water, q.s.	1000.00	ml.

Dissolve tris (hydroxy-methyl) amino-methane in approximately 150 ml. of distilled water. Add lactic acid and mix well. 10 N NaOH is added to the solution until it is alkaline as indicated by phenolphthalein. *Do not add phenolphthalein to solution.* This mixture is heated to about 80° C. to depolymerize the lactic acid. Cool; then add hydroxylamine hydrochloride and approximately 400 ml. of distilled water. Adjust pH to 7.6 with 10 N NaOH and bring to final volume of 1 L. with distilled water.

3. *0.00525 M NAD in 0.05 M Tris Buffer pH 7.6*

NAD	0.4 Gm.
Tris buffer, pH 7.6	232.0 ml.

Prepare sufficient NAD in buffer for the number of measurements to be made. Approximately 250 ml. is needed for thirty measurements of standards, tests and blanks.

Apparatus

The basic unit with a 37° C. heating bath in lieu of a dialyzer is used in this

LACTATE DEHYDROGENASE

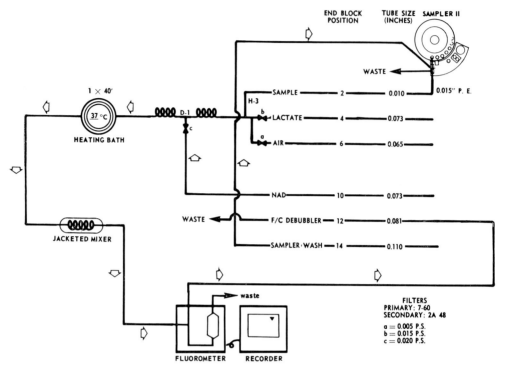

Fig. VI-3.—Flow diagram for lactate dehydrogenase.

procedure. In place of the colorimeter, a fluorometer with a general purpose UV lamp (360 mμ emission) is used.

Operating Notes

The standards are prepared fresh from a commercial "in-serum" laboratory control.* This "in-serum" control is reconstituted with distilled water, and serial dilutions are made. Blanks are run on all specimens by substituting tris buffer for the lactate substrate and resampling the specimens.

1. Turn the recorder module to "on" position by moving the top toggle switch upward. Do not turn chart drive on.

2. Turn fluorometer on by the toggle switch. Let warm up a few minutes, then press lamp button to activate the lamp. Let this stabilize for about 15 minutes.

3. Stretch manifold block to first or second notches and lock pump rollers on the platen. Pump water through the system for 10 to 15 minutes.

4. Switch reagent lines to proper reagents.

5. After about 5 minutes turn recorder chart drive on by means of lower toggle switch.

*Hyland Abnormal Chemistry Control Sera.

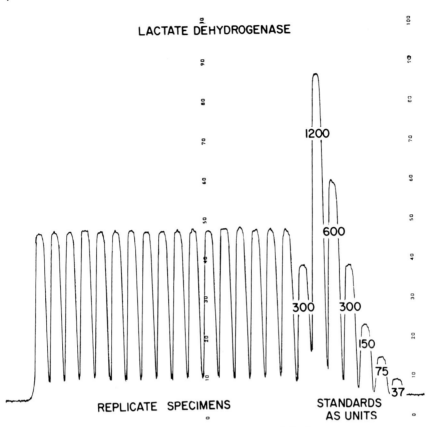

Fig. VI-4.—Recorder tracing for lactate dehydrogenase.

6. By means of blank dial on fluorometer, set reagent base line to desired setting (about 5 per cent T).

7. Place high standard on platter and aspirate. Adjust high standard peak to read between 85 and 95 per cent T. Then place standards and samples on platter for run. Situate platter on the sampler with first standard opposite sampling probe. Keep platter covered during sampling.

8. Aspirate the samples at the rate of 40/hr.

9. After the last sample has been recorded, substitute tris buffer for L-lactate and repeat sampling of specimens for test blanks.

10. When the last sample blank has been recorded, turn off the chart drive. Place all reagent lines in distilled water. Wash the system for at least 10 minutes or until all reagents have been washed from the system.

11. Release the rollers and manifold block.

Calculations

The results are read directly from the chart recordings.

GLUTAMIC OXALOACETIC TRANSAMINASE (GOT)

Principle

GOT activity is measured by coupling the transamination reaction to a secondary enzyme reaction in which one of the products, oxaloacetate, is reduced to malate by malate dehydrogenase. As $NADH_2$ is oxidized, the intensity of its fluorescence at 470 mμ, when excited by 340 mμ light, diminishes. The change in fluorescence is proportional to $NADH_2$ concentration and, hence, GOT activity.

Preparation of Reagents

1. *Stock Phosphate Buffer (pH 7.4)*

Potassium phosphate (mono basic)	136 Gm.
Sodium hydroxide	33 Gm.
Distilled water, q.s.	1000 ml.

Slowly dissolve the KH_2PO_4 in about 800 ml. of distilled water. Then add NaOH and allow to cool. Adjust pH to 7.4 and dilute to 1 L.

2. *Working Phosphate Buffer (pH 7.4)*

Stock Phosphate buffer	100 ml.
Distilled water, q.s.	1000 ml.

Dilute stock phosphate buffer to 1 L.

3. *0.15 Gm. Per Cent Albumin*

Stock phosphate buffer	50.00 ml.
Fraction V bovine albumin	0.75 Gm.
Distilled water, q.s.	500.00 ml.

Dilute stock phosphate buffer to 500 ml. with distilled water. Add albumin and mix gently until in solution. Mixture should be kept sealed in refrigerator.

4. *NADH$_2$ (.32 mg./ml.)*

NADH$_2$, 90 per cent	17.5 mg.
Albumin phosphate buffer, 0.15 Gm. per cent	50.0 ml.

Dissolve NADH$_2$ in albumin buffer. This solution should be kept in ice water bath and shielded from light. Prepare fresh daily.

5. *MDH (3 I.U./ml.)*

MDH, pig heart	as calculated below
Albumin phosphate buffer	0.15 Gm. per cent

Dilute malate dehydrogenase (MDH) with 0.15 Gm. per cent albumin buffer to give a concentration of 9 I.U./ml. The enzyme can be stored in freezer ($-20°$ C.) at least a month in convenient aliquots; on day of use thaw gently and dilute 1:3 with 0.15 Gm. per cent albumin solution for final conc. of 3 I.U./ml. Keep in ice water bath and shielded from light.

Example calculations for MDH preparation:

MDH in vial = 10 mg. total × 210 units/mg. = 2100 I.U./vial

$$\text{desire 9 I.U./ml., } \therefore \frac{2100}{9} = 233$$

Dilute entire vial to 233 ml. with 0.15 Gm. per cent albumin in PO$_4$ buffer, then freeze as 10 ml. aliquots ($-20°$ C.); when diluted to 30 ml. this amount will provide reagent sufficient for 100 to 120 minutes. Approximately 40 samples can be analyzed during this time.

6. *GOT Substrate*

Stock phosphate buffer	100.00 ml.
Sodium hydroxide, 1 N	128.00 ml.
L-aspartic acid	18.50 Gm.
α-ketoglutaric acid	2.63 Gm.
Distilled water, q.s.	1000.00 ml.

Dilute stock phosphate buffer to 800 ml. and mix well. Add 1 N NaOH followed by L-aspartic acid and α-ketoglutaric acid with thorough mixing. Adjust pH to 7.4 and bring to final dilution of 1 L.; add 0.5 ml. of chloroform and store in refrigerator. Bring to room temperature before using.

Apparatus

This method calls for a basic unit using a fluorometer with a general purpose UV lamp (360 mμ emission) as the sensing device and a heat bath for additional incubation.

Operating Notes

The standards are prepared fresh from a commercial "in-serum" laboratory control.[*] This "in-serum" control is reconstituted with distilled water, and appropriate dilutions are made.

---

[*]Hyland Special Chemistry Control Sera.

GLUTAMIC OXALOACETIC
AND
GLUTAMIC PYRUVIC TRANSAMINASE

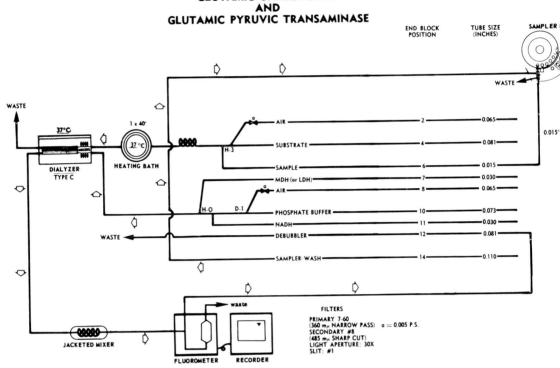

Fig. VI-5.—Flow diagram for GOT and GPT.

1. Turn the recorder module to "on" position by moving the top toggle switch upward. Do not turn chart drive on.

2. Turn fluorometer on by the toggle switch. Let warm up a few minutes, then press lamp button to activate the lamp. Let this stabilize for about 15 minutes.

3. Stretch manifold block to first or second notches and lock pump rollers on the platen. Pump water through the system for 10 to 15 minutes.

4. Switch reagent lines to proper reagents.

5. After about 5 minutes turn recorder chart drive on by means of lower toggle switch.

6. By means of blank dial on fluorometer, set reagent base line to desired setting (about 95 per cent T).

7. Place high standard on platter and aspirate. Adjust high standard peak to read between 10 and 20 percent T. Then place standards and samples on platter for the run. Situate platter on the sampler with first standard opposite sampling probe. Keep platter covered during sampling.

8. Aspirate the samples at the rate of 40/hr.

9. When the last sample has been recorded, turn off the chart drive. Place all reagent lines in distilled water. Wash the system for at least 10 minutes or until all reagents have been washed from the system.

10. Release rollers and manifold block.

Calculations

The results are read directly from the chart recordings.

GLUTAMIC PYRUVIC TRANSAMINASE (GPT)

Principle

$$
\begin{array}{ccccc}
\underset{\text{Alanine}}{\overset{\displaystyle\text{CH}_3 \;|\; \text{CHNH}_2 \;|\; \text{COO}-}{}} & + & \underset{\alpha-\text{ketoglutarate}}{\overset{\displaystyle\text{COO}- \;|\; \text{CO} \;|\; \text{CH}_2 \;|\; \text{CH}_2 \;|\; \text{COO}-}{}} & \underset{\displaystyle\longrightarrow}{\overset{\displaystyle \text{GPT}}{\rightleftarrows}} & \underset{\text{Pyruvate}}{\overset{\displaystyle\text{CH}_3 \;|\; \text{CO} \;|\; \text{COO}-}{}} + \underset{\text{Glutamate}}{\overset{\displaystyle\text{COO}- \;|\; \text{CHNH}_2 \;|\; \text{CH}_2 \;|\; \text{CH}_2 \;|\; \text{COO}-}{}}
\end{array}
$$

$$
\underset{\text{Pyruvate}}{\overset{\displaystyle\text{CH}_3 \;|\; \text{CO} \;|\; \text{COO}-}{}} + \text{NADH}_2 \; \underset{\displaystyle\longrightarrow}{\overset{\text{lactate}\atop\text{dehydrogenese}}{\rightleftarrows}} \; \underset{\text{Lactate}}{\overset{\displaystyle\text{CH}_3 \;|\; \text{CHOH} \;|\; \text{COO}-}{}} + \text{NAD}
$$

GPT activity is measured by coupling the transamination reaction to a secondary enzyme reaction in which one of the products, pyruvate, is reduced by lactic dehydrogenase. As $NADH_2$ is oxidized, the intensity of its native fluorescence diminishes. This change in fluorescence is proportional to $NADH_2$ concentration and, hence, GPT activity.

Preparation of Reagents

The basic reagents are the same as in the method for GOT. Alternate reagents for this method are as follows:

1. *LDH (39 I.U./ml.)*

LDH (rabbit muscle 2 × crystallized)	as calculated below
Albumin phosphate buffer	0.15 Gm. per cent

Dilute lactate dehydrogenase (LDH) with 0.15 Gm. per cent albumin buffer to give a concentration of 117 I.U./ml. The enzyme can be stored in the freezer ($-20°$ C.) at least a month in convenient aliquots. On day of use, thaw gently and dilute material 1:3 with 0.15 Gm. per cent albumin solution for final concentration of 39 I.U./ml. Keep in ice water bath and shielded from light. Example calculations for LDH preparation:

$$\text{LDH in vial} = 100 \text{ mg. total} \times 59 \text{ I.U./mg.} = 5900 \text{ I.U./vial}$$
$$\text{desire 117 I.U./ml: } \therefore \frac{5900}{117} = 50$$

Dilute entire vial to 50 ml. with 0.15 Gm. percent albumin in PO_4 buffer.

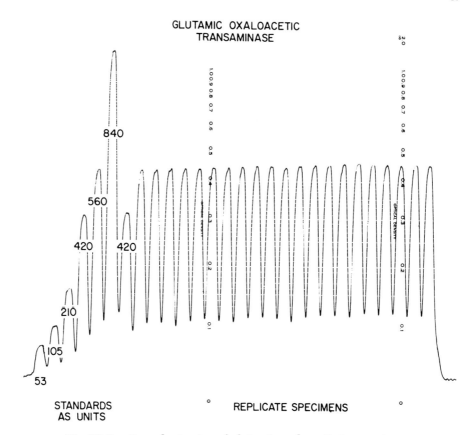

Fig. VI-6.—Recorder tracing of glutamic oxaloacetic transaminase.

Freeze as 10 ml. aliquots ($-20°$ C.); when diluted to 30 ml., this amount will provide sufficient reagent for 110 to 120 minutes. Approximately 40 samples can be analyzed during this time.

2. *GPT Substrate*

Stock phosphate buffer	100.00 ml.
1-alanine	27.70 Gm.
α-ketoglutaric buffer	1.73 Gm.
Distilled water, q.s.	1000.00 ml.

Dilute stock phosphate buffer to 800 ml. and mix well. Add 1-alanine and α-ketoglutaric acid. When the chemicals are in solution, adjust to pH 7.4 and bring to final dilution of 1 L. Add 0.5 ml. of chloroform and store in refrigerator. Bring to room temperature before using.

Apparatus

This method calls for a basic unit using a fluorometer with a general purpose UV lamp (360 mμ emission) as the sensing device and a heating bath for additional incubation.

Operating Notes

The standards are prepared fresh from a commercial "in-serum" laboratory control.* This "in-serum" control is reconstituted with distilled water, and appropriate dilutions are made.

1. Turn the recorder module to "on" position by moving the top toggle switch upward. Do not turn chart drive on.

2. Turn fluorometer on by the toggle switch. Let warm up a few minutes, then press lamp button to activate the lamp. Let this stabilize for about 15 minutes.

3. Stretch manifold block to first or second notches and lock pump rollers on the platen. Pump water through the system for 10 to 15 minutes.

4. Switch reagent lines to proper reagents.

5. After about 5 minutes turn recorder chart drive on by means of lower toggle switch.

6. By means of blank dial on fluorometer set reagent base line to desired setting (about 95 per cent T).

7. Place high standard on platter and aspirate. Adjust high standard peak to read between 10 and 20 per cent T, then place standards and samples on platter for run. Situate platter on the sampler with first standard opposite sampling probe. Keep platter covered during sampling.

8. Aspirate the samples at the rate of 40/hr.

9. When the last sample has been recorded, turn off the chart drive. Place all reagent lines in distilled water. Wash the system for at least 20 minutes or until all reagents have been washed from the system.

10. Release rollers and manifold block.

Calculations

The results are read directly from the chart recordings.

ACID PHOSPHATASE (Method of King-Armstrong)

Principle

Acid phosphatase activity is measured by the amount of phenol released from disodium phenyl phosphate at the selected pH of 4.9. Incubation is for one hour at 37° C. After hydrolysis, protein is precipitated with Folin-Ciocalteau reagent, and phenol is determined by measuring the blue color which is produced by the addition of sodium carbonate. The color is probably due to the formation of a "heteropoly blue" complex which results from treatment of phosphotungstate and phosphomolybdate with reducing agents, phenol in this instance.

A unit of acid phosphatase is defined as the enzymatic activity which will liberate 1 mg. of phenol from a 0.005 M solution of disodium phenyl phosphate in citrate buffer at pH 4.9 in 1 hr. at 37° C.

---

*Hyland Special Chemistry Control Sera.

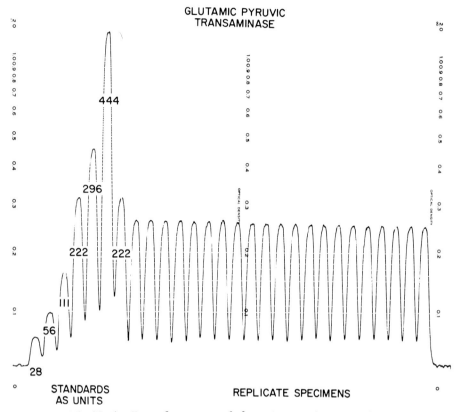

Fig. VI-7.—Recorder tracing of glutamic pyruvic transaminase.

Preparation of Reagents

1. *Phenol Reagent—(Harleco)*

| Folin-Ciocalteau phenol reagent | 1 part |
| Distilled water | 2 parts |

Dilute phenol reagent with distilled water and mix well.

2. *Disodium Phenol Phosphate Substrate (0.01 M)*

| Phenyl disodium phosphate | 2.18 Gm. |
| Distilled water, q.s. | 1000.00 ml. |

Dissolve the phenyl disodium phosphate in distilled water and dilute to final volume. Sterilize the solution by bringing it quickly to the boiling point. Cool it immediately, add a few drops of chloroform, and store in the refrigerator.

3. *Acid Buffer (pH 4.9)*

Citric acid, crystalline (monohydrate)	21 Gm.
Sodium hydroxide, 1N	188 ml.
Distilled water, q.s.	500 ml.

Dissolve the citric acid in 200 ml. of water. Add NaOH and dilute to volume. The pH of this solution should be 4.9. If necessary, adjust pH by addition of 1N HCl or 1N NaOH. Add a few drops of chloroform, and store in the refrigerator in a polyethylene bottle.

4. *Stock Phenol Standard (1 mg./ml.)*

Phenol	100 mg.
Hydrochloric acid, conc.	5 ml.
Distilled water, q.s.	100 ml.

The phenol plus the conc. HCl is diluted to final volume with distilled water.

5. *Buffered Acid Substrate*

Disodium phenylphosphate	250 ml.
Acid buffer	250 ml.

Mix substrate and buffer together, and store in the refrigerator in a polyethylene bottle.

6. *Sodium Carbonate, 0.8 Per Cent (W/V)*

Sodium carbonate, anhydrous	80 Gm.
Distilled water, q.s.	1000 ml.

Dissolve the carbonate in the distilled water and dilute to volume. Store in a polyethylene bottle.

7. *Standard Curve*

Prepare working standards as indicated in the chart below, and use 0.005 N HCl as the diluent to insure a shelf life of at least 2 months.

Concentration of Standard in mg. Per Cent	ml. of Stock Standard Required	Final Volume (ml.)
1	5	500
2	10	500
4	20	500
5	25	500
6	30	500
8	40	500
10	50	500

Apparatus

No special equipment is necessary for this test procedure. However, an accurate 37° C. heating bath is used. The final color production is read in a Coleman Jr. spectroscope at a wavelength of 660 mμ.

Procedure

Incubation and deproteinization:

1. Pipet 4.0 ml. of buffered acid substrate into each of two test tubes labeled "test" and "control" and allow to warm for 3 minutes in a 37° C. water bath.

2. Add 0.2 ml. of serum to the tube labeled "test," mix at once and replace in the water bath.

3. Exactly one hour after the addition of serum, add 2.0 ml. of diluted phenol reagent to both tubes and mix well.

4. Add 0.2 ml. of serum to tube marked "control," mix and centrifuge both tubes.

Colorimetric analysis:

1. Prepare a blank by mixing 4.0 ml. of buffered substrate, 0.2 ml. distilled water, and 2.0 ml. diluted phenol reagent in a test tube.

2. Prepare standards by mixing 1 ml. of the working phenol standard, 3.2 ml. of buffered substrate, and 2.0 ml. of diluted phenol reagent in a test tube. For a standard curve, use all of the working standards. Usually one standard, 0.05 mg./ml., is sufficient for determination of unknown once linearity and reproducibility of the method and reagents have been established.

3. To appropriately labeled 19 mm. cuvets, add 4.0 ml. of the supernatant of the unknowns and 4.0 ml. of the blank and standard dilutions.

4. To all cuvets, add 6.0 ml. of 8 per cent sodium carbonate and allow to stand for 20 minutes. Then read in Coleman spectrophotometer at 660 mμ.

Results and Calculations

Determine phenol concentration from a standard curve, or calculate the concentration from the absorbency of a standard of known concentration.

When working standard is used, calculate as follows:

$$\text{KA units} = \frac{\text{O.D. "Test"} - \text{O.D. "Control"}}{\text{O.D. "Standard"}} \times \frac{\text{Value of Standard}}{(0.05 \text{ mg./ml.})} \times \frac{100}{0.20}$$

AMYLASE

Principle

The blue color formed by the reaction of starch with iodine can be measured spectrophotometrically. The decrease of blue color, due to enzymatic digestion of starch after incubation, is a measure of amylase activity when compared with the unreacted control.

Preparation of Reagents

1. *Buffered Starch Substrate (pH 7.0)*

Disodium phosphate, anhydrous	26.60 Gm.
Benzoic acid	8.40 Gm.
Starch, Merck-Linter (soluble)	0.40 Gm.
Distilled water, q.s.	1000.00 ml.

Dissolve phosphate and benzoic acid in 500 ml. of water. Heat to boiling. Using an analytical balance, weigh-out and dissolve starch in 10 ml. of *cold* water. *Add the boiling buffer solution* to the starch, stirring constantly, and then boil for one minute. Cool and dilute to 1 L. with distilled water. This is stable at room temperature.

2. *Stock Iodine Solution*

Potassium iodate (KIO_3)	3.57 Gm.
Potassium iodide (KI)	45.00 Gm.
Hydrochloric acid, conc.	9.00 ml.
Distilled water, q.s.	1000.00 ml.

Add the KIO_3 and KI to 800 ml. of distilled water and mix. Add slowly while mixing the conc. HCl. Allow to cool and dilute to 1 L.

3. *Working Iodine Solution*

Potassium fluoride	25.0 Gm.
Stock iodine solution	50.0 ml.
Distilled water, q.s.	500.0 ml.

Add the fluoride to about 350 ml. of water and mix. Add the stock iodine, mix, and dilute to 500 ml. final volume. Store in a dark bottle. This solution is stable for one to two months if stored in the refrigerator.

Apparatus

The equipment used is standard and found in most clinical laboratories, and includes a 37° C. water bath and a Coleman Jr. spectrophotometer.

Operating Notes

1. Pipet 5.0 ml. of Linter starch substrate into each of two 50 ml. volumetric flasks marked "test" and "control."

2. Place the test flask in a water bath at 37° C. for 5 minutes to warm the contents. The control need not be incubated.

3. Pipet exactly 0.1 ml. of serum into the bottom of the test flask, gently mix and allow the reaction to proceed for exactly 7½ minutes at 37° C. water bath. NOTE: The serum should be delivered from a 0.1 ml. Mohr pipet or a micropipet with care to avoid contamination of specimen with saliva. No serum is added to the control.

4. After 7½ minutes, remove "test" flask from water bath.

5. Immediately add 5 ml. of working iodine solution to both flasks.

6. Dilute both flasks to 50 ml. with distilled water immediately and mix well.

7. Measure optical density of the "test" and "control" *without* delay against a water blank at 660 mμ.

Calculations and Results

$$\frac{\text{O.D. Control} - \text{O.D. Test}}{\text{O.D. Control}} \times 800 = \text{Units of Amylase}/100 \text{ ml. serum}$$

If the activity of amylase in the serum exceeds 400 units, the test is repeated using fivefold dilution of serum. The final result is calculated by multiplying by 5. Serum should be diluted with 0.9 Gm. per cent NaCl.

ALDOLASE

Principle

Aldolase is an enzyme normally found in small concentrations in the serum but in high concentrations in most tissues of the body, especially skeletal muscle. Aldolase catalyzes the following reaction:

$$\text{Fructose-1, 6-Diphosphate} \rightleftharpoons \begin{array}{c}\text{Dihydroxyacetone}\\\text{Phosphate}\end{array} + \begin{array}{c}\text{Glyceraldehyde-3-}\\\text{Phosphate}\end{array}$$

Hydrazine is present in the reaction mixture to combine with the products of a forward reaction which are called triose-phosphates. This prevents their disappearance due to other enzymes in the serum. The triose-phosphates are hydrolyzed at room temperature with alkali to the corresponding trioses which are then converted to "osazones" by the 2, 4-dinitrophenylhydrazine of the aldolase color reagent. On making the mixture alkaline, the characteristic color of osazones is formed. The ozone color intensity is proportional to the amount of triose present, while the amount of triose produced is related to the amount of aldolase present.

Preparation of Reagents*

1. Pipet 1 ml. of water into a 50 ml. erlenmeyer flask labeled "blank," pipet 1.0 ml. aldolase calibration solution (Sigma #750-11) into flask labeled "standard."

2. Add the following to both flasks in the order indicated and mix by swirling after each addition:

        0.1 ml. hydrazine solution (#750-3)
        1.0 ml. 10 per cent trichloracetic acid
        2.0 ml. 0.75 N NaOH
        2.0 ml. Aldolase color reagent (#750-2)

3. Place both flasks in water bath at 37° C. for 60 minutes. After 60 minutes, add 14.0 ml. 0.75 N NaOH. Mix well by swirling and leave at room temperature (25° ± 5° C.).

4. Pipet blank and standard solutions into 6 cuvets in the proportions shown in the following chart:

Cuvet No.	"Blank" ml.	"Standards" ml.	Optical Density	Equiv. to S-L Units Aldolase/ml. Serum
1	5.0	0	—	0
2	4.0	1.0	—	25
3	3.0	2.0	—	50
4	2.0	3.0	—	75
5	1.0	4.0	—	100
6	0	5.0	—	125

Record the wavelength used. Record the optical densities of cuvets #2 through 6 using cuvet #1 as reference at 540 mμ ± 40 mμ. The wavelength or filter used here must be used for all the aldolase determinations. All

---

*Reagents may be obtained as Sigma Kit 750, Sigma, St. Louis, Mo.

readings must be completed within 15 minutes after the addition of the sodium hydroxide in Step #3.

5. Record O.D. in the space provided in Column 4. Plot a calibration curve of your O.D. vs. the corresponding S-L units of aldolase shown in Column #5. The line will not necessarily be straight. NOTE: Although the actual procedure uses only 0.2 ml. serum, the curve obtained from this chart will yield the activity per full milliliter without further multiplication.

Apparatus

A Beckman DU or equivalent spectrophotometer is the only special equipment needed for this procedure.

Operating Notes

1. Label two test tubes "test" and "blank." Pipet 1.4 ml. tris buffer (Sigma #750-4), 0.2 ml. hydrazine sulfate solution (Sigma #750-3) and 0.2 ml. serum into both tubes and place into 37° C. bath to warm.

2. To "test" tube, add 0.2 ml. aldolase substrate solution (Sigma reagent A), shake gently to mix, and replace in the water bath. Record exact time reagent A is added.

3. After exactly 30 minutes, add 2.0 ml. of 10 per cent trichloroacetic acid (Sigma reagent G) to both tubes. Add 0.2 ml. of reagent A to "blank" tube. Shake both tubes to mix.

4. Centrifuge both tubes. Transfer 1.0 ml. of clear supernatant fluids to appropriately labeled cuvets which are clean and dry.

5. Add 1.0 ml. 0.75 N NaOH (Sigma reagent F) to each tube, mix gently and allow tubes to stand at room temperature for a minimum of 10 minutes but no longer than 20 minutes.

6. Add 1.0 ml. aldolase color reagent (Sigma #750-2), mix gently and place in 37° C. water bath. Record time.

7. After 60 minutes, remove tubes from the bath and add 7.0 ml. 0.75 N NaOH. Mix several times by inversion and allow to stand at room temperature (25° ± 5° C.) for 5 minutes (minimum).

8. Using the tube labeled "blank" as reference, read O.D. of the test in the same instrument and at the same wavelength as that used in preparing the calibration curve. Determine aldolase activity of the unknown from the calibration curve. If a value greater than 125 S-L units per ml. is obtained, repeat test using a fivefold serum dilution (1 part serum plus 4 parts water).

Unit Definition

One S-L (Sibley-Lehninger) unit of aldolase activity is the amount of enzyme which will split 1 milliliter of fructose-1, 6-diphosphate per hour at 37° C. under the assay conditions described in the procedure, i.e.,

$$\text{S-L} = \frac{1}{22.4} \ \mu \text{ moles of fructose-1, 6-diphosphate hydrolized per hour at } 37°\text{C.}$$

$$= \frac{2}{22.4} \ \mu \text{ moles of alkali-labile P formed per hour at } 37°\text{C.}$$

$$= \frac{62}{22.4} \ \mu\text{g alkali-labile P formed per hour at } 37°\text{C.}$$

CREATINE PHOSPHOKINASE (CPK)

Principle

The enzyme creatine-phosphokinase catalyzes the phosphorylation of creatine by ATP. This reaction is significant in heart and striated muscle tissue. Like other energy-producing phosphorus compounds, creatine-phosphate accumulates as reserve energy in the relaxed muscle; hence, the largest amount of creatine-phosphate can be found here. CPK exhibits greatest activity in striated muscle tissue, followed in turn by the brain and the heart. CPK activity in the serum is greatly increased in muscular disorders, such as progressive muscular dystrophy.

The enzyme creatine phosphokinase catalyzes the reversible reaction.

$$\text{creatine} + \text{ATP} \rightleftharpoons \text{creatine phosphate} + \text{ADP}$$

The activity of creatine phosphokinase is determined with creatine as substrate. The rate of increase of ADP formed per time unit is assayed in the auxiliary reaction which is catalyzed by pyruvate kinase.

$$\text{ADP} + \text{PEP} \rightleftharpoons \text{ATP} + \text{pyruvate and in the indicator}$$
reaction which is catalyzed by lactic dehydrogenase
$$\text{pyruvate} + \text{NADH}_2 + \text{H} + \rightleftharpoons \text{lactate} + \text{NAD}$$

The quantity of $NADH_2$ consumed in the above reaction per time unit can be measured spectrophotometrically.

Preparation of Reagents

Reagents are obtained in a kit; C. F. Bohebringer and Soehne, G.M.B.H., Creatine Phosphokinase Kit, UV method.

1. *Reduced Disphophopyridine Nucleotide/Adenosine-5′-Triphosphate/ Phosphophenolypyruvate in Glycine Buffer (NADH₂/ATP/PEP)*

2M glycine buffer, pH 9; $8 \cdot 10^{-4}$M $NADH_2$; $6 \cdot 10^{-3}$M ATP; $2 \cdot 10^{-3}$M PEP; $1 \cdot 10^{-2}$M $MgSO_4$
Dissolve contents of bottle (1) in 15 ml. of redistilled water.

2. *Lactic Dehydrogenase/Pyruvate Kinase (LDH/PK)*

2 mg. of enzyme protein/ml.
The suspension in bottle (2) will not be diluted.

3. *Glycine-Creatine Buffer (Buffer/Substrate)*

$1 \cdot 10^{-1}$M glycine buffer, pH 9; $6.3 \cdot 10^{-2}$M creatine
Dissolve contents of bottle (3) in 20 ml. of redistilled water.

Stability of solutions:
If kept tightly closed and if stored at 2 to 4° C., the dissolved substances from bottle will be stable for approximately two weeks. LDH/PK, buffer/substrate and buffer will be stable for at least six months, if kept at the same temperature. Since the buffer solutions may eventually absorb carbon dioxide from the air, keep bottles always tightly closed; verify pH after a certain period of time and adjust, if needed, with a few drops of concentrated NaOH.

Procedure

Run a blank for each sample and read against this blank. Pipet into each test tube:

Sample	Blank
1.00 ml. serum	1.00 ml. serum
0.70 ml. NADH$_2$/ATP/PEP (1)	0.70 ml. NADH$_2$/ATP/PEP (1)
0.05 ml. LDH/PK (2)	0.05 ml. LDH/PK (2)

Mix and allow to stand for 10 minutes at 25° C. 1.75 ml. buffer/substrate and 1.75 ml. buffer added to the "sample" and "blank" respectively; mix and transfer solutions into 10 mm. Beckman cells. Set the photometer at optical density of 0.300 at a wavelength of 340 mμ with the blank being placed into the light path, and read the optical density of sample against blank (O.D.$_1$). Exactly 10 minutes after the first reading, the blank is adjusted to 0.300 and the optical density of the sample is read against the blank (O.D.$_2$).

The difference in optical density (O.D.$_1$ − O.D.$_2$) = Δ O.D. − CPK is used for calculation. On account of very low CPK activities which are obtained with normal sera (e.g., at 366 mμ: Δ O.D. − CPK = 0.005), the precision of the measurement is limited by the stability of the photometer. Negative values for Δ O.D. − CPK may therefore be obtained.

If the difference in optical density exceeds 0.300/10 min. (more than 66 CPK units), dilute 0.20 ml. of serum with 1.80 ml. of 0.85 Gr. per cent saline solution and repeat assay. Correct for this tenfold dilution factor in the final calculations.

Apparatus

The only special equipment needed is a Beckman DU or equivalent spectrophotometer.

Calculations and Results

One unit is that amount of enzyme per ml. serum which at 340 mμ and 25° C. would cause a change in NADH$_2$ optical density of 0.001/min. in a 3 ml. assay volume.

Using 1.00 ml. of serum, and with a test volume of 3.50 ml. and a reaction period of 10 minutes, it thus follows that

$$\triangle \text{ O.D. } \frac{340 \text{ m}\mu}{\text{CPK}} \bullet 116 = \text{CPK units/ml. of serum}$$

REFERENCES

GENERAL

1. Howell, R. R.: The diagnostic value of serum enzyme measurements. J. Pediat. 68: 121–134, 1966.

2. Rymenant, M. V., and Tagnon, H. J.: Medical Progress: Enzymes in clinical medicine. New Eng. J. Med. 261:1325–1330, 1959.

3. Zinkham, W. H., Blanko, A., and Kupchyk, L.: Isozymes: Biological and clinical significance. Pediatrics. 37:120–131, 1966.

ALKALINE PHOSPHATASE

1. Bessey, O. A., Lowry, O. H., and Brock, M. B.: A method for the rapid determination

of alkaline phosphatase with five cubic millimeters of serum. J. Bio. Chem. 164:321–329, 1946.

2. Gutman, A. B.: Serum alkaline phosphatase activity in diseases of the skeletal and hepatobiliary systems. Amer. J. Med. 27:875–901, 1959.

3. Mabry, C. C., Gevedon, R. E., Roeckel, I. E., and Gochman, N.: Submicro automation of a central clinical chemistry laboratory. In Skeggs, L. T., Jr. (Ed.): Technicon Symposia 1966, Automation in Analytical Chemistry, New York, Mediad Press, Inc., 1967, pp. 18–28.

4. Morgenstern, S., Kessler, G., Auerbach, J., Flor, R. V., and Klein, B.: An automated p-nitrophenylphosphate serum alkaline phosphatase procedure for the autoanalyzer. Clin. Chem. 11:876–888, 1965.

LACTATE DEHYDROGENASE

1. Amador, E., Dorfman, L. E., Wacker, W. E. C.: Serum lactic dehydrogenase activity: An analytical assessment of current assays. Clin. Chem. 9:391–399, 1963.

2. Brooks, L., and Olken, H. G.: An automated fluorometric method for determination of lactic dehydrogenase in serum. Clin. Chem. 11:748–762, 1965.

3. Passen, S., and Gennaro, W.: An automated system for the fluorometric determination of serum lactate dehydrogenase; Its adaptability to an automated system for the simultaneous determination of both serum lactate dehydrogenase and serum glutamic oxalacetic transaminase. Amer. J. Clin. Path. 46:69–81, 1966.

TRANSAMINASES

1. Levine, J. B., and Hill, J. B.: Automated fluorometric determinations of serum glutamic oxalacetic transaminase and serum glutamic pyruvic transaminase. In Skeggs, L. T., Jr. (Ed.). Technicon Symposium; Automation in Analytical Chemistry. New York, Mediad, Inc., 1966, pp. 569–574.

2. Wilkinson, J. H.: Measurement of NAD Enzymes. In Sunderman, F. W. (Ed.): Applied Seminar on Laboratory Diagnostics of Liver Diseases. Philadelphia, Association of Clinical Scientists II:1966, pp. 1–11.

3. Wroblewski, F.: The clinical significance of transaminase activities of serum. Amer. J. Med. 27:911–923, 1959.

ACID PHOSPHATASE

1. King, E. J., and Armstrong, A. R.: A convenient method for determining serum and bile phosphatase activity. Canad. Med. Ass. J. 31:376–381, 1934.

2. King, E. J., and Armstrong, A. R.: Alkaline and acid phosphatase. In Reiner, M. (Ed.): Clinical Chemistry, vol. I. New York, Academic Press, Inc., 1953, pp. 75–83.

3. Klein, B., Auerbach, J., and Morgenstern, S.: Automated determination of acid phosphatase. Clin. Chem. 11:998–1008, 1965.

4. Woodard, H. Q.: The clinical significance of serum acid phosphatase. Amer. J. Med. 27:902–910, 1959.

AMYLASE

1. Caraway, W. T.: A stable starch substrate for the determination of amylase in serum and other body fluids. Amer. J. Clin. Path. 32:97–99, 1959.

2. Howell, R. R.: The diagnostic value of serum enzyme measurements. J. Pediat. 68:121–134, 1966.

ALDOLASE

1. Aronson, S. M., and Volk, B. S.: Studies on serum aldolase activity in neuromuscular disorders. Amer. J. Med. 22:414–421, 1957.

2. Sibley, J. A.: Significance of serum aldolase levels. Ann. N. Y. Acad. Sci. 75:339-348, 1958-1959.

3. Sibley, J. A., and Lehninger, A. L.: Aldolase in the serum and tissues of tumor-bearing animals. J. Nat. Cancer Inst. 9:303–309, 1948–1949.

4. Sibley, J. A., and Lehninger, A. L.: Determination of aldolase in animal tissues. J. Biol. Chem. 177:859–872, 1949.

5. Volk, B. W., Losner, S., Aronson, S. M., and Lew, H.: The serum aldolase level in acute myocardial infarction. Amer. J. Med. Sci. 232:38–43, 1956.

CREATINE PHOSPHOKINASE

1. Tazner, M. L., and Gilvarg, C.: Creatine and creatine kinase measurement. J. Biol. Chem. 234:3201–3204, 1959.

CHAPTER VII

Tolerance, Absorption, and Function Studies

GLUCOSE TOLERANCE

Clinical Annotation

THE CAPACITY of a person to dispose of ingested glucose is referred to as his glucose tolerance. Glucose tolerance tests and various modifications have been used since the beginning of the century for the diagnosis of diabetes. The assessment of a patient's reaction to a loading dose of glucose also is useful in detection of and understanding of a number of other metabolic disorders. To date, this test has been most used in the detection and in the management of diabetes mellitus. In the detection of various metabolic disorders, it has been underused; but, for the detection of diabetes, in our opinion, it has been overused. Other disorders in which the test may be useful include hypoglycemia, adrenal impairment, unexplained glycosuria, hepatic glycogen storage disease, malabsorption, and pheochromocytoma.

On those patients with overt diabetes, the response to a loading dose of glucose usually adds little to the understanding of the patient's disorder. But in those patients in whom the diagnosis of diabetes may be obscured, measuring their response to a glucose challenge is indispensable in establishing an early diagnosis of diabetes.

There is a high incidence of diabetes (3 to 5 per cent of the population when followed to old age), and the disorder is frequently associated with degenerative disorders. Thus, a simple and effective survey procedure for hospital and clinic patients, a high probability group, is desirable. Urine sugar results are quite variable and result in over-referrals for glucose tolerance tests. We suggest the one- or two-hour postprandial blood sugars as optimal periods for monitoring the patient's response to usual carbohydrate loads. A one- and a two-hour blood sugar of > 140 mg. per cent and > 120 mg. per cent, respectively, are suspicious of diabetes. Patients who have greatly elevated values do not need a glucose tolerance test for diagnosis of diabetes.

As a general rule, the glucose tolerance test is indicated when a diagnosis of diabetes cannot be definitely established or rejected and in the following types of patients, all of whom show a higher than ordinary tendency to diabetes.

1. Women who have delivered large babies or who have had pregnancies terminated by abortions, premature labor, stillbirths, or neonatal deaths.

2. Individuals who are obese.

3. Individuals with a family history of diabetes.

4. Individuals who were themselves large babies.

5. Patients with transitory glycosuria or nondiagnostic hyperglycemia, especially during the course of pregnancy, surgical procedures, trauma, emotional stress, myocardial infarction, cerebrovascular accident, or administration of adrenal steroids.

6. Patients with unexplained episodes of hypoglycemia.

7. Patients with otherwise unexplained neuropathy, retinopathy, nephropathy, peripheral vascular disease, or coronary artery disease.

The one-dose oral glucose tolerance test is the procedure used by most clinicians. There is no conclusive evidence that other tests are more accurate or more sensitive than the one-dose oral glucose tolerance test, which is still very much the "standard" for this purpose. However, the cortisone-modified glucose tolerance test used in conjunction with the one-dose glucose tolerance test does show some promise for even earlier detection of diabetes.

Procedure

The oral glucose tolerance test is performed as follows:

1. Maintain the patient on a diet with usual carbohydrate content (150 to 300 Gm. for adults and an equivalent lesser amount for infants and children) for at least three days preceding test.

2. An overnight fast of eight to ten hours precedes the test.

3. Blood and urine samples are taken before the test.

4. The oral loading of glucose is administered over several minutes in a dose dependent on age and body size. "Ideal" weight is used for obese patients. A 25 per cent solution flavored with noncaloric orange or lemon is practical.

Age	Dose
Up to 18 months	2.5 Gm./kg.
1½ to 3 years	2.0 Gm./kg.
3 to 12 years	1.75 Gm./kg.
Over 12 years	1.25 Gm./kg. (maximum 100 Gm. total dose)
Adults	100 Gm., total dose

5. Venous blood in adults and older children and capillary blood in infants and young children are taken, along with urine specimens, over a period of several hours. Suggested times for most patients are: fasting or zero, one-half hour, one hour, one and a half hours, two hours, three hours, and four hours. A five-hour specimen may be of value in assessing patients with hypoglycemia.

Collection Precautions

Serum, plasma, and blood have essentially the same sugar concentration. When blood is allowed to stand without preservative at room temperature, the glucose is utilized at an approximate rate of 5 per cent per hour. Thus, the specimen should either be refrigerated or the serum (plasma) removed shortly after it is obtained. Note should be made as to whether specimens were derived from venous or capillary (arterial) blood. Vomiting of the ingested glucose during the first hour will invalidate the results. The usual precautions for blood sugar collections as described earlier must be observed.

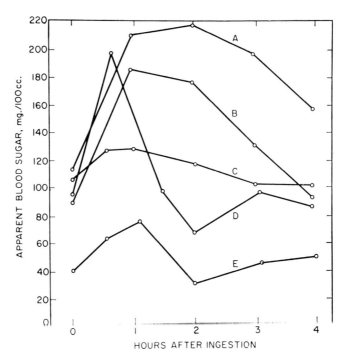

Fig. VII-1.—Oral glucose tolerance test. Five types of abnormal response. Hyper-glycemia unresponsiveness: A: diabetic type, B: hepatic type, C: malabsorption. Hyperglycemia over-responsiveness: D: functional hypoglycemia. Lacking hyper-glycemia: E: hyperinsulinism. (From Behrendt, H.: Diagnostic Tests in Infants and Children, ed. 2, Philadelphia, Lea and Febiger, 1962.)

Interpretation of Results

When glucose is administered on a weight basis, the younger child can dispose of the prescribed dose more effectively. Thus, the relative dose is larger in the younger child. There is a wide variation in the normal response, and representative abnormal responses are shown.

In interpreting the results of this test, it is necessary to become somewhat arbitrary. Using the procedure and doses we have described for the one-dose oral glucose tolerance test, the blood sugar and urine glycosuria results in our laboratory are usually interpreted as shown. For a patient to be designated "diabetic," two or more blood sugar levels as listed in the Diabetic column should occur. The physician must recognize that capillary blood gives 15 to 25 mg. per cent and 1 to 15 mg. per cent greater values when the venous blood is 160 mg. per cent and 120 mg. per cent respectively. At fasting and hypoglycemic levels, venous and capillary blood sugars are essentially the same.

STEROID MODIFIED GLUCOSE TOLERANCE

Clinical Annotation

This test, introduced in 1954, combines the demonstrated insulin antagonistic

Table VII-1.—Significance of One-Dose Oral Glucose Tolerance Test

Time	Normal	Latent Diabetic, Normal Variant, or Improper Testing	Diabetic
	Serum or Plasma (mg Per Cent)		
Fasting	90 (80–110)	110–120	>120
½ hr.	130 (100–140)	140–150	>150
1 hr.	150 (120–160)	160–170	>170
1½ hr.	130 (100–140)	140–150	>150
2 hr.	90 (80–110)	110–130	>130
3 hr.	90 (80–110)	110–120	>120
4 hr.	90 (80–110)	70–110	>110
Urine	No glycosuria	1–2 plus glycosuria on 1–2 specimens	2–4 plus glycosuria on 2 or more specimens

action of cortisone with the glucose tolerance test. The hope was that the added stress provided by cortisone-induced gluconeogenesis would bring out cases with relative deficiencies of insulin who would be likely to develop overt diabetes in the future. Subsequent reports have shown that it is useful in this respect, especially when testing the family and relatives of diabetics.

Procedure

As originally described, the procedure combined a one-dose oral glucose tolerance test with oral administration of 50 mg. (62.5 mg. of body weight > 160 lbs.) of cortisone at eight and a half and two hours prior to glucose loading. The blood sugar response was compared with an oral glucose tolerance test, using the same glucose load administered forty-eight hours earlier. There have been a number of modifications of the procedure, which seem allowable, since orally ingested cortisone has its maximal effect three to four hours after ingestion. However, since experience is limited, we are adhering to the original dose schedule with adaptations for children as follows:

Age/Size of Patient	Cortisone Dose, in Evenly Divided Doses, 8 1/2 and 2 Hours Preceding Second GTT
0–1 mo.	25 mg. (12.5 mg. × 2)
1 mo.–5 yr.	50 mg. (25 mg. × 2)
5 yr.–10 yr.	75 mg. (37.5 mg. × 2)
10 yr.–18 yr.	100 mg. (50 mg. × 2)
Adult < 160 lbs.	100 mg. (50 mg. × 2)
Adult > 160 lbs.	125 mg. (62.5 mg. × 2)

Interpretation of Results

The original investigators designated blood sugar values of 160 mg. per cent, 150 mg. per cent and 140 mg. per cent for the one, one and a half and two hour test periods respectively for deciding between normal and abnormal. Regardless of the values selected by these investigators or in subsequent studies by others, there is much overlap and lack of bimodality in the frequency distribution of the results. Thus, the values selected are arbitrary and follow-up observations are limited. Because our blood sugar method gives a slightly higher value than the older Somogyi-Nelson method, and since we do not want to report an excessive number of "false positive" latent diabetics, we use slightly higher "deciding" blood sugar levels than some investigators. We use the values of 180 mg. per cent, 170 mg. per cent, and 160 mg. per cent for the one, one and a half and two hour test periods, respectively, as the critical levels.

GALACTOSE TOLERANCE

Clinical Annotation

Galactose, an isomer of glucose, occurs free and complexed in many foods. When ingested, galactose reaches the liver where it is converted into glucose and stored as glycogen. Recognition of this liver function half a century ago initiated galactose tolerance testing. Today, with more discrete liver function tests available, galactose loading is used only when a specific defect in galactose metabolism is suspected. For galactosemia, galactose loading may be deleterious in that hypoglucosemia results. Thus, other forms of testing (erythrocyte gal-1-PO$_4$ uridyl transferase assay, sugar identification, response to galactose free diet, etc.) are preferred. Galactose loading tests are useful in evaluating patients with various forms of hepatic glycogen storage disease and in galactose malabsorption syndromes. In von Gierke's disease (glucose-6-phosphatase defect or Type I glycogen storage disease), galactose loading causes (1) no change in blood glucose, (2) an increase in blood lactate, and (3) a decrease in blood pH and CO$_2$ content. These changes and the rapid disappearance of galactose are due to galactose bypassing glycogenolysis. The same phenomena occur in these patients when fructose is administered. Patients with other forms of glycogen storage disease usually respond to galactose normally with a rise on blood glucose with no lactic acidosis.

Procedure

Patients are prepared as for an oral glucose tolerance test. A suitable loading dose schedule, using a 10 per cent galactose solution, is the same as for an oral one-dose glucose tolerance test, but with a maximum dose of 50 Gm. of galactose. The blood sugar response is measured at fasting or zero, one-half, one, one and a half, two, three, and four hours. When glycogen storage disease is suspected, lactic acid, blood pH, and total CO$_2$ measurements obtained on the same specimens are helpful in evaluating the patient.

Collection Precautions

The patient should be observed carefully throughout the test. A patient with galactosemia may develop hypoglucosemia leading to convulsions. A patient with glycogen storage disease may develop profound acidosis. The physician should be prepared to administer glucose and/or bicarbonate intravenously as indicated.

Interpretation of Results

In normal patients, the peak blood galactose level is reached at one-half to one hour, and the values are the same as or less than in the glucose tolerance test. In galactosemia, there is a greatly elevated and sustained rise in total blood sugar, most of which is galactose, with copious amounts of galactosuria. In hepatic glycogen storage disease, especially von Gierke's (I), there is a negligible rise (< 20 mg. per cent) in total blood sugar; the ingested galactose does not appear in the blood. In galactose malabsorption syndromes, there is a little increase (< 20 mg. per cent) in total blood sugar during the test period. When there is generalized liver damage, there is reduced tolerance with galactosuria.

DISACCHARIDE TOLERANCE

Clinical Annotation

Chronic diarrhea, due to deficient digestion and absorption of certain disaccharides, has been described recently in infants and adults both as congenital and acquired disorders. In these disorders, the incompletely digested carbohydrate is fermented by bacteria, leading to excretion of greatly increased amounts of short-chain organic acids in the feces. Also, ingested disaccharides appear in significant amount in the urine and feces following their ingestion. The clinical syndromes identified to date based on congenital intestinal disaccharidase deficit are: lactase (lactose) and combined sucrase-isomaltase (sucrose, isomaltose) deficiencies. The various disorders where diminished disaccharidase has been described on an acquired basis include: infectious diarrhea, sprue and celiac disease, cystic fibrosis, ulcerative colitis, regional enteritis, giardiasis, peptic ulcer, and postoperatively following upper small bowel resection.

Procedure

The patient is prepared as for a glucose tolerance test. In addition, he should be free of diarrhea for two to three days before the test. The disaccharide dose, as a 10 percent aqueous solution, is as follows:

Infants (0 to 2 yr.)	3 Gm./kg./body weight
Children (2 to 10 yr.)	2.5 Gm./kg./body weight
Older children and adults	2 Gm./kg./body weight
Maximum dose	100 Gm., total

Blood for sugar measurement is collected at fasting or zero time, one-half, one, one and a half, two, three, and four hours. The urine is collected over a five-hour period for sugar analysis. Stools are collected for twelve hours for pH and specific sugar analysis.

Interpretation of Results

Normally, the total blood sugar response is that of a one-dose oral glucose tolerance test. In the individual disaccharidase deficiency states, the total blood sugar curve is "flat" with little or no increase in concentration. Typically, disacchariduria and a large excess of the disaccharide in the stool can be detected. The stool pH, as examined with nitrazine paper, diminishes to pH 5.0 to 4.0 within six to eighteen hours. Inadequacy of digestion and absorption also is indicated by development of the symptoms of intestinal discomfort and diarrhea.

XYLOSE ABSORPTION

Clinical Annotation

The per cent excretion of d-xylose in urine after ingestion of a dose of d-xylose is used as an index of intestinal absorption. This pentose is not digested in the bowel, but is absorbed by diffusion. Over half of that absorbed is metabolized, the remainder being rapidly excreted in the urine. In malabsorption disorders involving primarily the small bowel, the amount that appears in the urine is diminished. Thus, normal values are found in pancreatic exocrine insufficiency and a variety of other digestive disturbances not affecting the bowel itself.

Procedure

The fasting child is given 10 ml./kg. body weight of a 5 per cent aqueous solution of d-xylose up to a maximum of 25 Gm.(500 ml.). The patient's bladder is emptied at the beginning of the test, and all urine passed during the five hours after ingestion is collected and pooled in one container; it is refrigerated or frozen until analyzed.

Collection Precautions

Suitable data is obtained only when the patient is well hydrated and voids two to three times during the test period. Inadequate urine volume usually results in a spuriously low recovery value.

Interpretation of Results

In adults, mean excretion is about 25 per cent of the ingested dose in normal subjects and about 10 per cent of the ingested dose in sprue or other primary malabsorptive disorders of the small bowel. There are no precise data for infants and children, so the test is most useful as a "screening" test. A recovery of less than 10 per cent of the test dose usually indicates a malabsoprtive defect.

GLUCAGON TOLERANCE

Clinical Annotation

Glucagon, a hormone secreted by the α cells of the pancreas, activates the hepatic phosphorylase system to cause glycogenolysis and the release of glucose from the liver. These phenomena occur only when there are both adequate glycogen stores and normal enzymes in the liver. The test is useful in studying patients with hepatic forms of glycogen storage disease or in excluding the diagnosis.

Procedure

The patient is fasted for six to ten hours, depending on the degree of hypoglycemia. Two control blood samples are obtained, then 30 μg glucagon per kilogram body weight, with a maximum of 1 mg., is administered intravenously. Blood is obtained for total sugar measurements at 15, 30, 45, 60, 90, and 120 minutes.

Interpretation of Results

Normally, a maximum rise in blood sugar of 25 to 100 mg. per cent or more than 50 per cent of control level occurs in 15 to 60 minutes, with a return to fasting levels within 60 to 90 minutes. If hyperglycemia does not occur, repeat the test two to three hours after a meal. Glucagon produces a poor blood sugar response, even after a good meal, in hepatic glucose-6-phosphatase (I), brancher enzyme (IV) and phosphorylase (VI) deficiencies. When no blood sugar rise occurs following a moderate fast, but does so moderately following a meal, hepatic debrancher (III) or synthetase (VII) enzymes may be deficient. The diagnosis of the type of glycogen storage disease may be inferred following these tests, but responses are variable and new forms of glycogen storage disease are being described as shown. Exact diagnosis can only be established by biochemical analysis of liver biopsy material.

EPINEPHRINE TOLERANCE TEST

Epinephrine (1) activates the phosphorylase system in muscle, fat, and liver; (2) inhibits the peripheral uptake of glucose; and (3) increases glycogenolysis in muscle. Because of the nonspecificity and multiple effects, the epinephrine tolerance test has been replaced by the glucagon tolerance test. It is performed, as is the glucagon tolerance test, by using epinephrine in a dose of 0.03 mg./kg. intramuscularly, not exceeding 0.3 mg. The blood sugar responses are similar to those of glucagon.

LEUCINE TOLERANCE TEST

Clinical Annotation

Leucine, an amino acid naturally occurring in protein, stimulates the release of insulin from the β cells of the pancreas. This results in a lowering of the blood glucose level. In the normal individual, the lowering of the blood glucose level is minimal and transient. In some individuals with hypoglycemia including some with islet cell adenomas, a profound and acute lowering of blood glucose occurs, which may result in hypoglycemic convulsions.

Procedure

The dose of L-leucine is dissolved in a small amount of warm water; 2.43 Gm./100 ml. at 25° C. is the limit of solubility. After a short fast, 150 mg./kg. body weight is given by mouth or nasogastric tube over a 2 to 5 minute period.

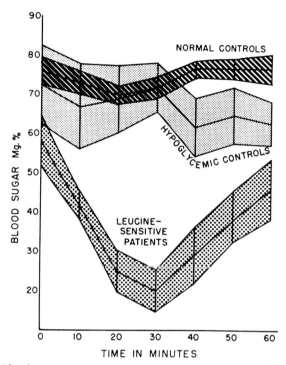

Fig. VII-2.—Blood sugar responses to intravenous 1-leucine. (From Mabry, C. C., DiGeorge, A. M., and Auerbach, V. H.: Leucine-induced hypoglycemia. J. Pediat. 57:526–538, 1960.)

Two control blood samples and individual ones at 15, 30, 45, 60, 90, and 120 minutes after oral leucine are obtained for sugar measurement. For intravenous testing, the chromatographically pure L-leucine is dissolved in isotonic saline, autoclaved to insure sterility, and administered intravenously at a dose of 75 mg./kg. over a 1 to 2 minute period with blood specimens for sugar measurement obtained at 10 minute intervals for 1 hour.

Collection Precautions

The physician should be prepared to interrupt the test with intravenous 10 per cent glucose should the patient develop signs of hypoglycemic shock or convulsions.

Interpretation of Results

In the "sensitive" subject, there will be a blood sugar decline of at least 50 per cent of the fasting level. The initial blood sugar should be > 40 mg. per cent in order to monitor the change adequately. The blood sugar returning to near starting levels at one to two hours aids the confirmation of leucine sensitivity. This degree of sensitivity has been observed in infants and children with idiopathic hypoglycemia, in about half of the patients with islet cell adenomas tested, and in individuals pretreated with sulfonylureas and insulin.

TOLBUTAMIDE TOLERANCE TEST

Clinical Annotation

Tolbutamide provokes the secretion of insulin from the beta cells of the pancreas. In proper dosage an acute, but transient, decline in blood sugar results. The test is useful in studying patients with (1) preclinical diabetes, (2) hypoglycemia, and (3) in differentiating between diabetes and the hyperglycemic response to glucose which is found in some patients with obesity or hepatic insufficiency.

Procedure

For detection of diabetes, the test is performed after an overnight fast. Patients with hypoglycemia should be fasted for only two to four hours; the initial blood sugar level must not be too low to render testing hazardous and the results difficult to interpret. After a control blood specimen is obtained, 20 mg. of sodium tolbutamide per kilogram (for children) is injected intravenously over a 1 to 2 minute period. Additional blood specimens are obtained at 20, 30, 40, 60, 90, and 120 minutes for blood sugar measurement. For adults 1 Gm. of sodium tolbutamide is administered.

Interpretation of Results

A normal response consists of a fall in blood sugar 20 to 50 per cent below the fasting level within 20 to 30 minutes, with a return to near the initial level by 90 to 120 minutes. In infants and young children, the depth of depression is at 20 minutes; in older individuals the nadir occurs at 30 minutes. In patients with diabetes and preclinical diabetes, the blood sugar decline following tolbutamide is diminished, and the nadir occurs at 40 minutes. Exaggerated or profound hypoglycemic responses occur in instances of an islet cell adenoma and may or may not occur in leucine-sensitive hypoglycemia. In other forms of hypoglycemia, the response is usually normal.

AMMONIUM CHLORIDE TOLERANCE TEST

Clinical Annotation

The kidney plays a major role in maintaining the body fluid ionic structure and optimal pH. In large part, this is done by multiple processes of recovery of basic radicals from the glomerular filtrate. Important components of this base preservation process include: (1) excretion of excess acid radicals, (2) excretion of predominately $H_2PO_4^-$ ions in lieu of HPO_4^-, (3) excretion of carbonic acid buffered radicals, and (4) ammonia formation. Ammonia formation in conserving base occurs as follows: If one chloride ion were to be filtered by the glomerulus, it would not proceed down the renal tubule as Cl^-. A cation such as sodium would be a requisite accompaniment of the anion. The kidney makes available for excretion ammonia, a weak base, which in the presence of an anion can become the cation, ammonium. The kidney thereby excretes one molecule of ammonium chloride, and the sodium ion remains (or is conserved) in the serum to continue to act as a base. This process is regulated by the degree of acid excess. Ammonium chloride loading probes the adequacy of the ammonia producing mechanism.

Procedure

The patient continues on a regular diet and fluid intake. A twenty-four hour urine is collected under mineral oil in an iced container. Two ml. concentrated HCl is added to prevent bacterial growth during collection and storage; urea splitting bacteria that produce ammonia must be suppressed. Immediately following this control period, the patient is administered NH_4Cl as a flavored aqueous solution in divided oral doses at six-hour intervals. A suggested dose schedule is as follows:

10 pound infant	1.5 Gm. NH_4Cl/day
20 pound infant	2.0 Gm. NH_4Cl/day
40 pound child	4.0 Gm. NH_4Cl/day
60 pound child	6.0 Gm. NH_4Cl/day
Adult	10.0 Gm. NH_4Cl/day

The patient is carefully observed and the test terminated if signs of acidosis become apparent. Twenty-four hour urine specimens are collected during the three-day test period; the collection precautions exercised for the control urine are used for the test urines. Also, a total plasma CO_2 and blood pH are collected at the end of each twenty-four hour period.

Interpretation of Results

Normal individuals respond to this dose of NH_4Cl by (1) increasing their ammonia production by not less than 75 per cent of the chloride increment and (2) decreasing their urine pH, to usually between 5 and 6, due to an increase in titratable acidity (organic acids). When tubular function is impaired, ammonia excretion is markedly reduced in the presence of adequately increased chloride excretion. If the tubular defect also involves loss of the ability to produce an acid urine, the pH will be close to the neutral point. Most patients with base-losing tubular disease show defects of both mechanisms, often in addition to other tubular deficiencies. Some of these disorders include renal tubular acidosis, de Toni-Fanconi syndrome, pan-nephritis, and cystinosis.

MEASUREMENT OF URINE AMMONIA
AND TITRATABLE ACIDITY

Principle

Titratable acidity is the total acid present in a twenty-four hour specimen expressed in terms of 0.1 N NaOH equivalents. It is measured by titration of the urine to neutrality with 0.1 N NaOH using phenolphthalein as an indicator. Urine ammonia is determined by Nesslerization.

Table VII-2.—Responses to Ammonium Chloride

	Before Test (Control)	Normal (3rd Day)	Affected Patient (3rd Day)
Blood:			
CO_2	normal	normal to slight decline	decline $10+$ mEq./L
pH	normal	slight decline	decline $0.1+$
Urine:			
NH_3	10–20 mEq./24	50–100 mEq./L.	10–20 mEq./L
Titratable acidity		greatly increased	little or no change
Na		little or no change	greatly increased
pH		$+$ to 4–5	remains 6–8

Reagents

1. *0.1 N Sodium Hydroxide*

   Sodium hydroxide, 1N   10 ml.
   Distilled water, q.s.   100 ml.

   Dilute sodium hydroxide with water and mix well. Store in a poly-ethylene bottle.

2. *Phenolphthalein, 1 Per Cent Solution*

   Phenolphthalein   1 Gm.
   Ethyl alcohol, 45 per cent   100 ml.

   Dissolve phenolphthalein in ethyl alcohol.

3. *Potassium Oxalate, Finely Pulverized*

4. *Nessler's Solution (Folin and Wu)*

   a. *Solution A*

   Potassium iodide   150 Gm.
   Iodine (I_2)   100 Gm.
   Mercury (Hg)   150 Gm.
   Distilled water, q.s.   100 ml.

   Mix ingredients in a 500 ml. volumetric flask for 7 to 15 minutes or until I^2 has nearly disappeared. Cool in running water until solution becomes pale red, and continue vigorous shaking until it becomes a greenish color. Decant solution and wash remaining Hg with water. Dilute solution plus the washings to 2 L. with distilled water.

   b. *Solution B; Sodium Hydroxide, 10 Per Cent*
   Sodium hydroxide   50 Gm.
   Distilled water, q.s.   500 ml.

   Dissolve sodium hydroxide in distilled water and dilute to volume.

   c. *Working Nessler's*
   Solution A   150 ml.
   Solution B   500 ml.
   Distilled water, q.s.   150 ml.

Mix well. It is preferable to allow this reagent to age for at least three weeks before use.

5. *Gum Ghatti*

| Gum ghatti, finely powdered | 0.5 Gm. |
| Distilled water, q.s. | 1000.0 ml. |

Heat about 700 ml. of water to about 70° C. Add the gum ghatti and stir with magnetic stirrer. Filter, dilute to 1 L., and add 0.5 ml. saturated alcoholic mercuric chloride. Store at room temperature.

6. *Stock Ammonia Standard (100 mg. Ammonia N/1)*

| Ammonium sulfate | 471.6 mg. |
| Distilled water, q.s. | 1000.0 ml. |

Dissolve $(NH_4)_2 SO_4$ in distilled water and dilute to volume.

7. *Working Standard*

| Stock standard | 1 part |
| Distilled water, q.s. | 19 parts |

Mix well stock standard and water.

Procedures for Ammonia and Titratable Acidity

1. Measure total volume of twenty-four hour specimen as milliliters.
2. For the ammonia determination prepare test, blank and standard tubes according to the following table:

	Urine	Water	Working Standard	Gum Ghatti	Nesslers Reagent
Test	0.2 ml.	1.8 ml.		2 ml.	0.8 ml.
Standard			2 ml.	2 ml.	0.8 ml.
Urine blank	0.2 ml.	4.6 ml.			
Reagent blank		2.0 ml.		2 ml.	0.8 ml.

Read in a spectrophotometer at 470 mμ using the reagent blank to set 0 optical density.

3. To determine titratable acidity:

Mix the specimen thoroughly. Pipet 25 ml. into a small flask and add a few drops of 1 per cent phenolphthalein. Add 10 Gm. of finely pulverized potassium oxalate. Shake well. Using 0.1 N NaOH, titrate to a permanent afint pink color. Record the milliliters of 0.1 N NaOH used for the titration.

Results and Calculations

Calculate the ammonia as follows:

$$\frac{\text{O.D. test} - \text{O.D. urine blank}}{\text{O.D. standard}} \times \text{value of standard} = \text{Ammonia in mEq./L.}$$

Calculate total acidity as follows:

$$\text{Total acidity} = \begin{array}{c} \text{ml. of 0.1 N NaOH} \\ \text{used in titration} \end{array} \times \frac{\text{ml. urine in 24 hr. specimen}}{\text{ml. urine in 24 hr. specimen}}$$

ENDOGENOUS CREATININE CLEARANCE

Clinical Annotation

Plasma creatinine is filtered through the glomeruli and passed unresorbed into the urine. Thus, its clearance gives an estimate of the glomerular filtration rate. Some tubular excretion may occur when plasma concentration of creatinine is high. Since in (1) normal individuals the endogenous creatinine clearance is almost identical with that of inulin, and (2) the test is easy to perform, it is practical for general use. In glomerular disorders, the endogenous creatinine clearance is diminished.

Procedure

1. The patient continues on a standard diet, but avoids tea or similar diuretic fluids. Adequate urine flow is most essential when a short urine collection period is used.

2. The bladder is emptied, and an accurately timed urine collection is made. These may be from one to twenty-four hours. Traditionally, toluene is used (1 to 3 ml.) as a preservative and the collection bottle is kept in the refrigerator until sent to the laboratory. We find that when clean collection bottles are used and the twenty-four hour specimen is delivered to the laboratory promptly, preservatives and cool storage do not alter the results. Precise timing to the closest minute is more critical than the duration of the collection.

3. At the end of the collection period, 2 ml. of fasting venous blood is drawn for creatinine content measurement.

4. Creatinine clearance may be altered by activity, so the patient should rest during the test. For prolonged urine collection, no excessive exercise is sufficient precaution.

Calculation

Endogenous creatinine clearance is expressed in ml. per minute and is corrected to the average adult surface area of 1.73 M^2 as follows:

$$\frac{U \times V}{P} \times \frac{1.73}{SA} = \text{ml./min.}$$

U is urine creatinine in mg./100 ml.
P is plasma creatinine in mg./100 ml.
V is urine volume in ml./min.
SA is surface area in square meters.
Normal values:
Newborn and premature infants   40-65 ml./min./1.73 M$_2$
Children
      males   124 ± 26* ml./min./1.73 M^2
      females   109 ± 14 ml./min./1.73 M^2
Adults
      males   105 ± 14 ml./min./1.73 M^2 (72–141)†
      females   95 ± 18 ml./min./1.73 M^2 (74–130)*

---

*S.D.
†Range

REFERENCES

GLUCOSE

1. Behrendt, H.: Carbohydrate metabolism tests. *In* Diagnostic Tests in Infants and Children, ed. 2. Philadelphia, Lea and Febiger, 1962, pp. 51–87.

2. Conn, J. W.: Interpretation of glucose tolerance test. Amer. J. Med. Science. 199: 555–564, 1940.

3. Cornblath, M., Wybregt, S. H., and Baens, G. S.: Studies of carbohydrate metabolism in the newborn infant: VII. Tests of carbohydrate tolerance in premature infants. Pediatrics. 32:1007-1024, 1963.

4. Hecht, A., Weisenfeld, S., and Goldner, M. G.: Factors influencing oral glucose tolerance; experience with chronically ill patients. Metabolism. 10:712–723, 1961.

5. Loeb, H.: Variations in glucose tolerance during infancy and childhood. J. Pediat. 68:237–242, 1966.

6. Mosenthal, H. O., and Barry, E.: Criteria for and interpretation of normal glucose tolerance tests. Ann. Intern. Med. 33:1175–1194, 1950.

STEROID MODIFIED GLUCOSE

1. Carrington, E. R., Shuman, C. R., and Reardon, H. S.: Evaluation of the prediabetic state during pregnancy. Obstet. Gynec. 9:664–669, 1957.

2. Conn, J. W.: The Banting Memorial Lecture, 1958. The prediabetic state in man; definition, interpretation and implications. Diabetes. 7:347–357, 1958.

3. Conn, J. W., and Fajans, S. S.: The prediabetic state: A concept of dynamic resistance to a genetic diabetagenic influence. Amer. J. Med. 31:839–850, 1961.

4. DiGeorge, A. M., and Moroney, J. D.: Cortisone modified glucose tolerance tests in children with fibrocystic disease of the pancreas. Personal communication.

5. Fajans, S. S., and Conn, J. S.: An approach to the prediction of diabetes mellitus by modification of the glucose tolerance test with cortisone. Diabetes. 3:296–304, 1954.

6. Fajans, S. S., and Conn, J. W.: The early recognition of diabetes mellitus. Ann. N. Y. Acad. Sci. 82:208-218, 1959.

7. Klimt, C. R., Wooff, F. W., Silverman, C., and Conant. J.: Calibration of a simplified cortisone glucose tolerance test. Diabetes. 10:351–366, 1961.

GALACTOSE

1. Anderson, C. M., Kerry, K. R., and Townley, R. R. W.: An inborn defect of intestinal absorption of certain monosaccharides. Arch. Dis. Child. 40:1–6, 1965.

2. Bruck, E., and Rapoport, S.: Galactosemia in an infant with cataracts. Amer. J. Dis. Child. 70:267–276, 1945.

3. Lindquist, B., Meeuwisse, G., and Melin, K.: Glucose-galactose malabsorption. Lancet. 2:666, 1962.

4. Marks, F., Norton, J. B., and Fordtran, J. S.: Glucose-galactose malabsorption. J. Pediat. 69:225–228, 1966.

5. Mason, H. H., and Turner, M. E.: Chronic galactemia. Report of case with studies of carbohydrates. Amer. J. Dis. Child. 50:359–374, 1935.

6. Schneider, A. J., Kinter, W. B., and Stirling, C. E.: Glucose-galactose malabsorption; report of a case with autoradiographic studies of a mucosal biopsy. New Eng. J. Med. 274:305–312, 1966.

DISACCHARIDE

1. Holzel, A., Schwarz, V., and Sutcliffe, K. W.: Defective lactose absorption causing malnutrition in infancy. Lancet. I:1126–1128, 1959.

2. Littman, A., and Hammond, J. B.: Progress in gastroenterology: Diarrhea in adults caused by deficiency in intestinal disaccharidases. Gastroenterology. 48:237–249, 1965.

3. Townley, R. R. W.: Review article: Disaccharidase deficiency in infancy and childhood. Pediatrics. 38:127–141, 1966.

XYLOSE

1. Benson, J. A., Jr., Cluver, P. J., Ragland, S., Jones, C. M., Drummey, G. D., and Bougas, E.: The d-xylose absorption test in malabsorption syndromes. New Eng. J. Med. 256: 335–339, 1957.

2. Butterworth, Jr., C. E., Perez-Santiago, E., de Jesus, J. M., and Santini, R.: Studies on the oral and parenteral administration of d (+) xylose. New Eng. J. Med. 261:157–164, 1959.

3. Fowler, D., and Cooke, W. T.: Diagnostic significance of d-xylose excretion test. Gut. 1:67–70, 1960.

4. Hadorn, V. B., Shmerling, D. H., and Blackert, R.: Der d-xylose-resorptionstest Helv. Paediat. Acta. 19:496–505, 1964.

5. Wolfish, M., Hildick-Smith, G. J., Ebbs, J. H., Connell, M. L., and Sass-Kortsak, A.: D-xylose tolerance test; a measure of intestinal absorption in normal and dystrophic infants. (Abstract) Amer. J. Dis. Child. 90:609–910, 1955.

GLUCAGON

1. Hug, G.: Glucagon tolerance test in glycogen storge disease. J. Pediat. 60:545–549, 1962.

2. Perkoff, G. T., Parker, V. J., and Hahn, R. F.: The effects of glucagon in three forms of glycogen storage disease. J. Clin. Invest. 41:1099–1105, 1962.

3. Cornblath, M., Ganzon, A. F., Demetrios, N., Baens, G. S., Hollander, R. J., Gordon, M. H., and Gordon, H. H.: Studies of carbohydrate metabolism in the newborn infant: III. Some factors influencing the capillary blood sugar and the response to glucagon during the first hours of life. Pediatrics. 27:378–389, 1961.

LEUCINE

1. Becker, F. O., Clark, J., and Schwartz, T. B.: L-leucine sensitivity and glucose tolerance in normal subjects. J. Clin. Endocr. 24:554–559, 1964.

2. Cochrane, W. A., Payne, W. W., Simpkiss, M. J., and Woolf, L. I.: Familial hypoglycemia precipitated by amino acids. J. Clin. Invest. 35:411–422, 1956.

3. DiGeorge, A M., Auerbach, V. H., and Mabry, C. C.: Elevated serum insulin associated with leucine-induced hypoglycemia. Nature (London). 188:1036–1037, 1960.

4. DeGeorge, A. M., and Auerbach, V. H.: Leucine-induced hypoglycemia; a review and speculations. Amer. J. Med. Sci. 240:792–801, 1960.

5. DiGeorge, A. M., Auerbach, V. H., and Mabry, C. C.: Leucine-induced hypoglycemia. III. The blood glucose depressant action of leucine in normal individuals. J. Pediat. 63: 295–302, 1963.

6. Fajans, S. S., Knopf, R. F., Floyd, Jr., J. C., Power, L., and Conn, J. W.: The experimental induction in man of sensitivity to leucine hypoglycemia. J. Clin. Invest. 42:216–229, 1963.

7. Floyd, Jr., J. C., Fajans, S. S., Knopf, R. F., and Conn, J. W.: Evidence that insulin release is the mechanism for experimentally induced leucine hypoglycemia in man. J. Clin. Invest. 42:1714–1719, 1963.

8. Floyd, Jr., J. C., Fajans, S. S., Conn, J. W., Knopf, R. F., and Rull, J.: Stimulation of insulin secretion by amino acids. J. Clin. Invest. 45:1487–1502, 1966.

9. McArthur, L. G., Kirtley, W. R., and Waife, S. O.: Effects of large doses of 1-leucine in animals and man. Amer. J. Clin. Nutr. 13:285–290, 1963.

10. Mabry, C. C., DiGeorge, A. M., and Auerbach, V. H.: Leucine induced hypoglycemia: I. Clinical observations and diagnostic considerations. J. Pediat. 57:526–538, 1960.

TOLBUTAMIDE

1. Cornblath, M., and Schwartz, R.: General considerations. In Schaeffer, A. J. (Consult. Ed.): Disorders of Carbohydrate Metabolism in Infancy. Philadelphia, W. B. Saunders, 1966, pp. 193–213.

2. Cunningham, G. C.: Tolbutamide tolerance in hypoglycemic children. Amer. J. Dis. Child. 107:417–423, 1964.

3. DiGeorge, A. M., and Chiowanich, P.: The intravenous tolbutamide response test in infants and children. Diabetes (Suppl.). 11:135–137, 1962.

4. Fajans, S. S., Schneider, J. M., Schteingart, D. E., and Conn, J. W: The diagnostic value of sodium tolbutamide in hypoglycemic states. J. Clin. Endocr. 21:371–386, 1961.

5. Kaplan, N. M.: Tolbutamide tolerance test in carbohydrate metabolism evaluation. Arch. Intern. Med. 107:212–224, 1961.

6. Unger, R. H., and Madison, L. L: A new diagnostic procedure for mild diabetes mellitus. Evaluation of an intravenous tolbutamide response test. Diabetes. 7:455-461, 1958.

AMMONIUM CHLORIDE

1. O'Brien, D., and Ibbott, F. A.: Urine ammonia by nesslerization. In Laboratory Manual of Pediatric Micro- and Ultramicro- Biochemical Techniques, ed. 3. New York, Harper & Row, Publishers, Inc., 1962, pp. 34–35.

2. Seiverd, C. E.: Titratable acidity. In Chemistry for Medical Technologists, ed. 3. St. Louis, C. V. Mosby Co., 1958, p. 193.

3. Talbot, N. B., Sobel, E. H., McArthur, J. W., and Crawford, J. D.: Figure 20 in Functional Endocrinology. Cambridge Mass., Harvard University Press, 1952, p. 96.

CREATININE CLEARANCE

1. Tobias, G. J., McLaughlin, Jr., R. F., and Hopper, Jr., J.: Endogenous creatinine clearance; A valuable clinical test of glomerular filtration and a prognostic guide in chronic renal disease. New Eng. J. Med. 266:317–323, 1962.

CHAPTER VIII

Endocrine Tests

A VARIETY OF endocrine disorders are observed in children, some of which are unique to pediatric patients. Therefore, emphases and interpretations are different from those of adult endocrinology. For the most part, the methods of assay and measurement of individual hormones or their derivatives are accomplished by conventional means. When urine is the biologic fluid studied, there usually is no need for a "micro" procedure.

The special needs for the diagnosis and treatment of the child with an endocrine disorder are most apparent with certain endocrine function or reserve tests. Thus, the emphasis of this chapter is on the medication and collection schedules of selected function studies and on some newly modified laboratory procedures. The function tests presented are suitable for performance in the clinic or hospital ward; the laboratory procedures are reasonable for a central clinical laboratory. For an extensive description of most endocrine tests and procedures, the reader is directed to several compendia.

A. PITUITARY

Clinical Annotation

Seven known hormones (FSH, LH, MSH, TSH, ACTH, STH, and prolactin) are produced by the anterior pituitary. These pituitary hormones act directly on the body cells or on other endocrine glands to affect almost every organ. The gland itself is under control of the hypothalamus and is reciprocally affected by the hormones produced by other endocrine glands. The posterior lobe of the pituitary is part of a functional unit, known as the neurohypophysis, which includes portions of the hypothalamus. The neurohypophysis produces antidiuretic and oxytocic hormones.

Diminished or enhanced secretion of one or more of these pituitary hormones may occur. The degree of the abnormalities cannot be fully appreciated without laboratory confirmation. Some childhood disorders involving individual pituitary hormones are shown in tabular form.

Pituitary Tests

1. *Adrenal Corticotrophic Hormone (ACTH) Reserve.* Cortisol is the physiologic inhibitor of ACTH secretion in the usual feedback mechanism. A heightened blood level of cortisol shuts off ACTH secretion and a diminished blood level provokes the pituitary secretion of ACTH. Metyrapone (Metopirone®), in appropriate dosage, inhibits 11-β-hydroxylation in the adrenal cortex, thereby interfering with normal production of hydrocortisone. The fall in cortisol levels then normally causes a pituitary discharge of ACTH which in

Table VIII-1.—Selected Pituitary Hormone Alterations in Children

Hormone	Excess	Deficiency
Growth hormone (STH)	Eosinophilic adenoma	Hereditary disorders Congenital defects Destructive lesions of pituitary
Thyrotropin (TSH)	Athyreotic cretinism Goitrous cretinism Thyroiditis Iodine deficiency	Associated with congenital defect of STH Acquired destructive lesions of pituitary
Cortotropin (ACTH)	Cushing's syndrome Primary Addison's disease	Exogenous cortisone and derivatives Destructive lesions of pituitary Assoc. with cong. defect of STH or STH and TSH
Follicle-stimulating hormone (FSH)	Primary gonadal failure (Turner's or Klinefelter's syndromes)	Assoc. with cong. defect, usually with STH, STH and other trophic hormones Destructive lesions of pituitary
Interstitial cell stimulating hormone (ICSH or LH)	——	Destructive lesions of pituitary
Melanocyte stimulating hormone (MSH)	Addison's disease Lipoatrophic diabetes	Hereditary defect
Antidiuretic hormone (ADH)	——	Destructive lesions of pituitary Destructive lesions of pituitary
Oxytocic hormone	——	Destructive lesions of pituitary
Premature onset of gonadotrophic hormones (FSH, ICSH, LH)	Isosexual precocious puberty	——

turn stimulates the adrenal cortex to secrete large amounts of 11-deoxycortisol (compound S). This is measureable in the urine by the Porter-Silber method as either 17-hydroxycorticoids or 17-ketogenic steroids. Compound S has little or no inhibitory effect on ACTH output and has relatively weak glucocorticoid biologic activity.

Procedure

Day 1: Collect control urine over twenty-four hour period.

Day 2: Administer Metopirone® orally:

Adults	750 mg. q4h × 6 doses
Children > 60 lbs.	500 mg. q4h × 6 doses
Children < 60 lbs.	250 mg. q4h × 6 doses

Collect twenty-four hour urine.

Day 3: Collect twenty-four hour urine.

Measure 17-ketogenic steroids in the separate daily urine collections. Normally, 17-ketogenic steroid excretion increases 50 to 600 per cent. Failure to do so indicates anterior ptiuitary inability to secrete ACTH.

2. *Thyroid-Stimulating Hormone (TSH) Reserve.* A deficiency of TSH can produce all the characteristic features of hypothyroidism. A dormant but otherwise normal thyroid gland can be stimulated into activity by TSH, thus permitting one to distinguish between primary and secondary thyroid failure. The response is measured by changes in ^{131}I uptake by the thyroid gland and serum protein-bound iodine levels.

Procedure

1. Obtain serum protein bound iodine (PBI) and 24-hour ^{131}I thyroid uptake.

2. Allow about one week to elapse so that no radioactivity remains.

3. Administer TSH, intromuscularly, q 12 h × 4 doses.
    Adults 10 USP units/dose
    Children 10 USP units/dose
    Infants 5 USP units/dose

4. When TSH administration is completed, repeat 24-hour ^{131}I uptake and serum PBI.

In normal subjects TSH produces an appreciable increase in radioactive uptake and serum PBI level. In hypothyroidism due to primary thyroid gland failure, ^{131}I uptake and serum PBI remain low. In hypothyroidism due to pituitary failure, there is a significant rise in ^{131}I uptake and a slower rise in serum PBI.

3. *Antidiuretic Hormone Tests.* In patients with polydipsia and polyuria without glycosuria or azotemia, the differential diagnosis usually is between impaired production of antidiuretic hormone (ADH or vasopressin), congenital unresponsiveness of the renal tubule to vasopressin, and psychogenic polydipsia or compulsive water drinking. The functional state of the neurohypophysial-renal system may be evaluated by serial tests, including intravenous hypertonic saline and vasopressin under constant water-loading conditions. Volumes, specific gravity, and osmolarity of timed urines are measured.

Procedure

Discontinue all antidiuretic therapy until there is a full return of the polydipsia and polyuria; free access to water may be allowed. Thirty minutes after hydration has started with 20 ml. water/kg. orally, urine specimens are collected at 15 minute intervals measuring urine flow in ml./minute. An indwelling catheter should be used in order that timing may be precise. After copious urine flow is established (>15 ml./min. in adult, but proportionately less in infants and children), 3 per cent sodium chloride is given at the rate of 0.25 ml./kg. min. for 45 minutes. If no decrease in urine flow occurs during the infusion period or during a subsequent hour, then 0.1 unit vasopressin is given intravenously. Urines are collected every 15 minutes; the volumes, specific gravities, and osmolarities are measured. Potential responses to these tests are shown.

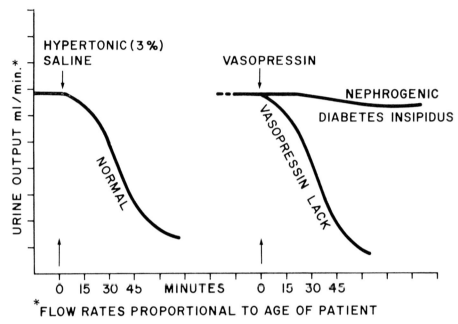

Fig. VIII-1.—Urine volume responses in diabetes insipidus.

B. ADRENAL

Clinical Annotation

The adrenal gland is composed of two independent portions, the cortex and medulla, which are quite different in structure and function. The cortex secretes a number of steroid compounds that can be grouped into several categories. The medulla, derived from ectoderm and sympathetic ganglia, secretes catecholamines.

CORTEX

1. *Glucocorticoids.* These have a 21-carbon structure with an —OH group in the 17 position and are referred to as 17-hydroxycorticosteroids. The principal steroid is hydrocortisone. The rate of corticosteroid production is under control of pituitary adrenocorticotropin (ACTH). These steroids have carbohydrate regulatory and anti-inflammatory properties. They and their metabolites are excreted in the urine and measured chemically as 17-ketogenic steroids or 17-hydroxycorticoids.

2. *Mineralcorticoids.* The principal steroid in this group is aldosterone. Its secretion is regulated only to a minor degree by pituitary corticotropin. Sodium deprivation is a much more potent stimulus to aldosterone secretion. Aldosterone controls sodium reabsorption in the distal tubules of the kidney, thus maintaining electrolyte equilibrium and stabilizing blood volume and blood pressure. It is excreted in the urine and can be measured only with difficult techniques.

Table VIII-2.—Selected Primary Adrenal Cortical Function
Disorders in Children

Disorder	Urine Measurement/Day		
Cortex:	17-Ketogenic Steroids	Aldosterone	17-Ketosteroids
1. Congenital adrenal hyperplasia — 5 forms (defect in steroidogenesis)	↓	±	↑
2. Cushing's syndrome	↑	N	N
3. Aldosteronism, primary (congenital or tumor)	N	↑	N
4. Aldosteronism, secondary (nephrosis, heart failure, etc.)	N	↑	N
5. Tumors	↑ or N	↑ or N	↑ or N
6. Addison's disease	↓	↓	N or ↓
7. Adrenal injury or aplasia	↓ or N	↓ or N	↓ or N

3. *Androgens.* These hormones promote growth and masculinization. They are capable of increasing retention of nitrogen, potassium, phosphorus, and sulfate. In the male, they are largely responsible for development of secondary sex characteristics. In the female, they are partly responsible for development of axillary and pubic hair. Metabolized adrenal androgens are excreted in the urine as 17-ketosteroids. In prepubertal children the urinary excretion of 17-ketosteroids is scant, but there is a constant increase throughout adolescence until adult levels are reached. In females all 17-ketosteroids are derived from the adrenals, while in the male about two-thirds is adrenal in origin, the remaining one-third being of testicular origin.

4. *Estrogens.* A small amount of these feminizing hormones are derived from the adrenal cortex.

MEDULLA

Principal catecholamines are norepinephrine and epinephrine, norepinephrine in larger amounts than epinephrine. Both hormones have pressor effects, norepinephrine accomplishing this without changing cardiac output. The major derivatives of catecholamines in urine are vanillylmandelic acid (VMA), metanephrine, and noremetanephrine. These are measured separately.

Normal adults excrete less than 100 μg of total free catecholamines/24 hr. The hospitalized patient or any person under stress may excrete up to 150 μg/24 hr. This is at variance with some published normal values, but we feel it more truly reflects the changes seen in our patients.

Patients with pheochromocytoma usually excrete greater than 500 μg/24 hr., and levels of several thousand micrograms are not uncommon.

Normal adults excrete up to 7 mg. of VMA/24 hr. As with catecholamines, hospitalized patients and other patients under stress may excrete up to 10 mg./24 hr. without sympatho-adrenal tumors.

Adrenal Tests

1. *Water Excretion Test.* This simple screening test is based on the observation that patients with adrenal cortical insufficiency excrete large amounts

Table VIII-3.—Pathologic Alterations in Total Catecholamines
and VMA Excretion

Increased Excretion	Decreased Excretion
Pheochromocytoma	Familial dysautonomia
Neuroblastoma	Transection of cervical spin cord
Ganglioneuroblastoma	Malnutrition
Ganglioneuroma	
Retinoblastoma	
Carotid body tumor	
Malignant carcinoid	
Heart disease (mild increase)	
Uremia (mild increase)	

Table VIII-4.—Alterations in VMA Excretion Due to Medication or Diet*

Increased Excretion	No Influence	Decreased Excretion
Bananas	α-Methyl-DOPA	Chlorpromazine
Epinephrine	Amphetamine	Iproniazid
Insulin shock	Citrus fruits	Morphine
Norepinephrine	Coffee	Pentobarbital
Reserpine (acute)	Ephedrine	p-Hydroxy-anphetamine
Salicylates	Glucose diet	Phenelzine
Selected tranquilizers	Guanethidine	Reserpine (chronic)
Histamine	Isopropylarternol	Imipramine
	Meprobamate	Segontin
	Angiotensin	

*Urine must be maintained at a pH less than 3 by the addition of 10 ml. of conc. HCl to the collection container.

Table VIII-5.—Total Free Catecholamine and VMA Urinary Excretion by Children

Age (years)	Catecholamines* (μg/24 hr.)	VMA (mg/24 hr.)
0–1	10–15	0.2–1.3
1–5	15–40	0.4–3.0
6–15	20–80	1.0–4.0
15–Adult	30–100	2.0–7.0

*Norepinephrine is usually excreted in much larger amount than epinephrine.

of sodium chloride in their urine so that their urine remains fairly concentrated despite ingestion of a large quantity of water. The effect is due to the stimulating effect of cortisol on renal glomerular filtration.

Procedure

1. Administer no corticosteroid medications for two days prior to test.

2. Add no salt to meals the day preceding the test.

3. In the morning after an overnight fast, have patient empty his bladder. Discard this urine.

4. Immediately thereafter give patient an oral load of water, 20 ml./kg. over 15 to 20 minutes.

5. During the next four hours, the urine is collected each hour and saved in labeled bottles.

Normally, 75 per cent of the water load is excreted during the subsequent four hours, the largest amount during the second hour. Patients with adrenal insufficiency excrete 50 per cent or less of the ingested water. The procedure can be repeated the following day, two hours after an oral dose of cortisone. (Adults 100 mg.; children 50 mg.; infants 25 mg.) If this corrects the lack of diuresis, primary adrenal cortical disease is likely.

2. *ACTH Stimulation Test.* This test estimates functional cortisol reserve. Urinary 17-ketogenic steroids are measured following stimulation of the adrenal cortex by intravenously administered ACTH.

Procedure

A control twenty-four hour urine is collected the day before the test. On the next three days, ACTH in saline is administered intravenously over an eight-hour period each day.

> Adults 40 units ACTH in 500 ml. 0.9 per cent NaCl
> Children 20 units ACTH in 250 ml. 0.9 per cent NaCl
> Infants 10 units ACTH in 100 ml. 09. per cent NaCl

Twenty-four hour urines are collected continuously for these three days.

Normally there is a three- to five-fold increase in urinary 17-hydroxycorticoids on the first day of the test with further small increases on successive days. Patients with Addison's disease show no increase in 17-hydroxycorticoids, whereas patients with pituitary ACTH deficiency will show an immediate response. Patients with Cushing's disease show a greatly exaggerated response.

C. THYROID

Synthesis of thyroxine, from tyrosine and iodide, is the function of the thyroid gland. The control of the gland by the anterior pituitary, which is partly under the control of the hypothalamus, is mediated via thyroid stimulating hormone (TSH). An excess of TSH results in hypertrophy and hyperplasia of the thyroid cells with increased collection of iodine and synthesis of thyroxine. TSH production is inhibited by the thyroxine secreted, and TSH production is activated in states of decreased thyroid hormone production. The gland secretes thyroxine into the circulation where it is associated with two globulin fractions that bind it specifically, as well as a minor fraction bound to prealbumin. Binding of thyroxine is not complete, however, and a very small fraction of the circulating thyroxine exists in the free, unbound state. It is this fraction that is thought to be the metabolically effective moiety in plasma.

Alterations in any of these physiologic states or hormone fractions may result in excess or deficient amounts of metabolically active thyroid hormone. It is essential in normal growth and maturation, water and mineral metabolism, protein and muscle metabolism, and lipid metabolism. Some childhood thyroid disorders and their effect on test results are tabulated.

TESTS

1. *Total Serum Organic Iodine* (Protein Bound Iodine, PBI)

Table VIII-6.—Selected Thyroid Function Disorders in Children

Disorder	PBI	BEI	^{131}I Uptake	T_3	Thyroid Autoantibodies
Congenital aplasia	→	→	→	→	0 – ±
Inborn error of thyroid synthesis, goitrous cretin, (5 forms)	↓, N, ↑	↓, N, ↑	↑, N	→	0
Acute thyroiditis	Variable	→	→	Variable	±
Chronic thyroiditis	Usually ↓	Usually ↓	→	→	+
Adolescent goiter	N	N	←	N	0
Graves disease	←	←	←	←	±
Iodine want (simple goiter)	N, ↓	N, →	←	N	0
Nephrosis and other states associated with plasma protein loss	→	→	—	←	0

Clinical Annotation

The protein bound iodine (PBI) has become the index laboratory test for measurement of thyroid gland function. The active hormones of the thyroid gland are unique in that they contain several iodide ions as an integral part of their molecules. Circulating hormone is almost entirely bound to specific proteins, collectively called thyroid binding proteins (TBP). Therefore, one is able to estimate thyroid hormone levels by determining the amount of iodine bound to protein, ie., PBI. A patient with excessive amounts of thyroid hormone therefore has an elevated PBI, while a patient who is producing less than normal amounts of hormone has a decreased PBI. The total serum organic iodine is a measure of the iodine content following removal of inorganic iodine from the serum. Since only trace amounts of organic iodine are not protein bound, the automated organic iodine values are nearly the same as PBI values.

Collection Notes

A venous blood sample is collected in iodine-free glassware. Vacutainers® are notably free of iodine contamination. Of course, preparation of the venipuncture site with iodinated disinfectants is contraindicated. Serum is used.

Interpretation of Results

The normal level of total serum organic iodine, as seen in 95 per cent of normal adults, is 3.5 to 9.6 μg/100 ml. The upper level of normal for total organic iodine is greater than the upper level of normal, 8.0 mg./100 ml., for PBI. At birth, the total organic iodine and PBI levels of the infant approximate that of the mother's. These values increase during the first week of life to 10 to 15 μg/100 ml. The levels then gradually decrease, but do not reach the levels of older children for several months. In children there is a cyclic change in serum organic iodine levels. The mean levels in late infancy are about 6.5 μg/100 ml.; they drop to a low mean level of about 5 μg/100 ml. during adolescence. The level then gradually rises to normal adult levels. There is a good correlation between results obtained with the automated acid distillation total organic iodine method we use and the clinical condition of the patient. However, there is an occasional patient in whom the correlation between the total serum organic iodine and the protein-bound iodine is not good.

METHOD

Principle

The automated procedure measures total serum organic iodine. Inorganic iodine is removed from the individual specimens prior to analysis by mixing with an anion exchange resin. The unabsorbed portions of the sera are aspirated into a digestor, and the organic matter is destroyed by heating with sulfuric acid in the presence of an oxidizing mixture of nitric and perchloric acids. This is accomplished in a rotating spiral glass vessel with controlled temperatures of 456° C. and 350° C. in two heating stages. The digestion of the sample is accomplished in 3 minutes as the sample is carried along the spiral grooves of the heated helix. The digest is analyzed for iodine by its catalytic effect on the reduction of ceric ion by arsenious acid. The concentration of iodine is proportional to the decrease in yellow ceric color. This is accomplished by adding water to the acid digest as it emerges from the second heating stage and aspirating an aliquot of the diluted digest into the output manifold. This aliquot is joined by an air-segmented stream of arsenious acid, mixed, and passed through a double heating coil for about 8 minutes. Finally, this effluent is passed through a flowcell colorimeter with 410 mμ filters.

Preparation of Reagents

1. *Anion Exchange Resin*

    Iobeads® Resin (Technicon Formula AR-150-65), Technicon Instruments Corp., Ardsley, New York.

2. *Sulfuric Acid, Conc.*

    Use concentrated analytical reagent (Baker's® preferred).

3. *Digestion Mixture*

Nitric acid, conc.	50. ml.
Perchloric acid, 70 per cent	200. ml.

    Add $HClO_4$ to HNO_3 carefully. Slight warming will occur. Mix well then transfer contents to an amber glass bottle. Prepare fresh each week.

4. *Arsenious Acid (0.2 N in 1N H_2SO_4)*

Arsenic trioxide	19.6 Gm.
Sodium hydroxide	14.0 Gm.
Sodium chloride	50.0 Gm.
Sulfuric acid, conc.	>56.0 ml.
Distilled water, q.s.	2000.0 ml.

    Dissolve the As_2O_3 and NaOH in approximately 200 ml. of water, using a 2 L. volumetric flask. When completely dissolved, dilute to about 800 ml. with more water. Add a few drops of phenolphthalein indicator; then add concentrated H_2SO_4 until the pink color is just discharged. Add an additional 56 ml. concentrated H_2SO_4. Dilute to 2 L. Add the NaCl and dissolve, then transfer to a polyethylene bottle and label.

5. *Ceric Ammonium Sulfate (0.01 N in 2N H_2SO_4)*

Ceric ammonium sulfate	6.3 Gm.
Sulfuric acid, conc.	52.0 ml.
Distilled water, q.s.	1000.0 ml.

    Dissolve the Ce $(HN_4)_4$ $(SO_4)_4 \cdot 2H_2O$ and concentrated H_2SO_4 in about 700 ml. water in a 1 L. volumetric flask. Allow to stand overnight, then dilute to volume with water. Filter through glass wool. Transfer to a polyethylene bottle and label.

**PROTEIN-BOUND IODINE
INPUT MANIFOLD**

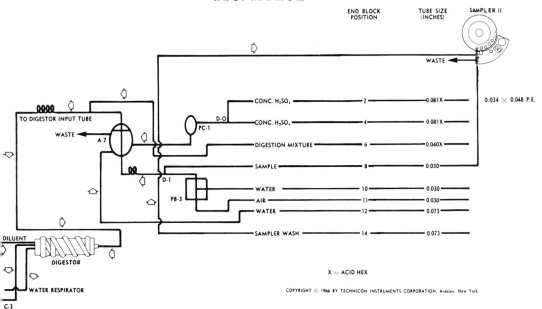

Fig. VIII-2.—Predigestor flow diagram for total organic iodine. (Copyright by Technicon Instruments Corporation.)

6. *Stock Iodate Standard (100 μg I/ml.)*

   Potassium iodate   16.85 mg.
   Distilled water, q.s.   100.00 ml.

   Dissolve KIO_3 in distilled water and dilute to volume.

   NOTE: *Do not use potassium iodide* for preparation of standards. Iodide can be absorbed from aqueous solution by the sample cup surface.

7. *Dilute Stock Iodate Standard (1 μg I/ml.)*

   Stock iodate standard   10 ml.
   Distilled water, q.s.   1000 ml.

   Add stock iodate standard to a 1 L. flask with distilled water and dilute to volume.

8. *Working Iodate Standards*

   Mix dilute stock iodate standard with distilled water according to the following table.

ml. Dilute Stock Iodate	Dilute to:	Resulting Concentrations of Working Standards μg I/100 ml.
5	200 ml.	2.5
5	100 ml.	5.0
10	100 ml.	10.0
15	100 ml.	15.0
20	100 ml.	20.0

PROTEIN–BOUND IODINE
OUTPUT MANIFOLD

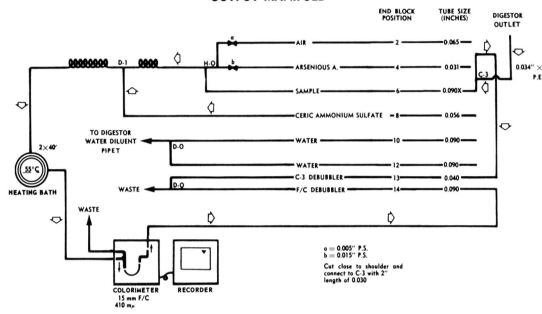

COPYRIGHT © 1966 BY TECHNICON INSTRUMENTS CORPORATION, Ardsley, New York

Fig. VIII-3.—Postdigestor flow diagram for total organic iodine. (Copyright by Technicon Instruments Corporation.)

Apparatus

The equipment used is shown in the flow diagram.

Operating Notes

A. *Contamination Check.*

Rationale: Grossly elevated levels of iodine (25 μg/100 ml. or more) are often encountered in the sera of patients who have recently received iodine-containing medicinals or roentgenographic contrast medias. To avoid contaminating the analytical system, a rapid screening of sample is carried out, using only a few microliters of the individual serum specimens.

Procedure

1. Turn on water aspirator full force.
   Turn on digestor.
   Turn on both proportioning pumps with all lines in water.
   Turn on recorder and colorimeter.
2. Set zero and 100 per cent T on recorder. Pump water for 10 minutes.
3. Put lines from input manifold #1 in reagents and sample line in water.
4. Pump reagents in manifold #1 for 10 minutes.

5. Turn on digestor heat. Set first heating at 1 ampere; second heating stage at 6 amperes.

6. Heat for 30 minutes.

7. Start reagents in output manifold #2. Base line should read between 10 per cent T and 20 per cent T.

8. Screen samples at 120/hr. Use special cam for this. Samples are compared with a 100 mcg. std. followed by three-water samples. Put water sample between each unknown sample.

9. After last sample has been recorded, turn heat off on digestor and remove Helix cover.

10. Turn off recorder.

11. Remove reagent lines from output manifold #2 and place in water.

12. Continue pumping reagents from input manifold #1 for 10 to 15 minutes while digestor is cooling.

13. Put reagent lines from input manifold #1 in water, continue pumping for 15 minutes to wash system out.

14. Turn off colorimeter.

Open proportioning pumps and release end blocks.

Turn off digestor pump.

Turn off aspirator.

Explanation of Rapid Scanning

Using the 120/hr. cam provided for scanning and a chart speed of 18 in./hr., a sample appears every 0.15 in. on the chart. The first and last cups of the screening procedure contain a 100 μg/100 ml. aqueous standard; these serve as markers for the run since only greatly contaminated specimens produce a peak. Identification of the contaminated specimen is facilitated by a scale with a mark at every 0.15 in. Grossly contaminated specimens are not suitable for analysis; do not attempt to analyze them.

B. *Preparation of Sample (Removal of Inorganic Iodine)*

Rationale: Traditionally, protein bound and inorganic iodine have been separated by protein precipitation and subsequent washing. This process has now been simplified by an inorganic resin which "traps" inorganic iodine.

Procedure

1. Transfer 1.5 to 2 ml. of serum to an iodine free, clean, dry test tube e.g., 16 mm. × 150 mm.

2. Pour approximately 300 mg. of Iobeads resin into the test tube.

3. Agitate continuously for approximately 5 minutes. A group of tubes may be placed in a mechanical shaker.

4. Allow resin to settle. Decant supernatant serum as soon as possible into the sample cup. Keep Iobeads out of cup to avoid clogging the sample line.

C. *Measurement of Total Organic Iodine*

Following the contamination check and the resin preparation, the individual seras are ready for automated measurement of their iodine content.

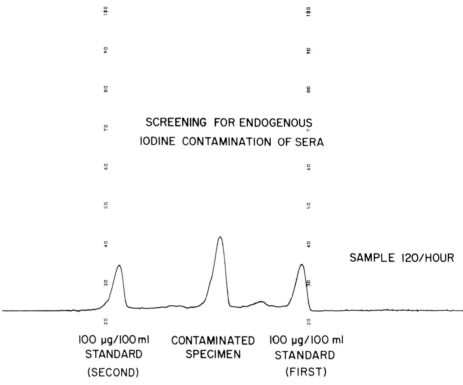

Fig. VIII-4.—Recorder tracing for contamination check prior to total organic iodine measurement.

Procedure

1. Turn on water aspirator full force.
   Turn on digestor.
   Turn on both proportioning pumps with all lines in water.
   Turn on recorder and colorimeter.

2. Set zero and 100 per cent T on recorder. Pump water for 10 minutes.

3. Put lines from input manifold #1 in reagents and sample line in water.

4. Pump reagents in manifold #1 for 10 minutes.

5. Turn on digestor heat. Set first heating at 1 ampere; second heating at 6 amperes.

6. Heat for 30 minutes.

7. Start reagents in output manifold #2. Base line should read between 10 per cent T and 20 per cent T.

8. Run resin treated sampler at 20/hr. using cam designed for this rate.

9. These samples are run along with a set of 5 standards: 2.5 μg/100 ml., 5 μg/100 ml., 10 μg/100 ml., 15 μg/100 ml., 20 μg/100 ml.

10. Put one-water sample after 20 μg/100 ml. standard.

11. Following the last sample, run another set of standards.

12. Run a PBI pool control and BEI pool control. These pool controls are treated just as just unknowns.

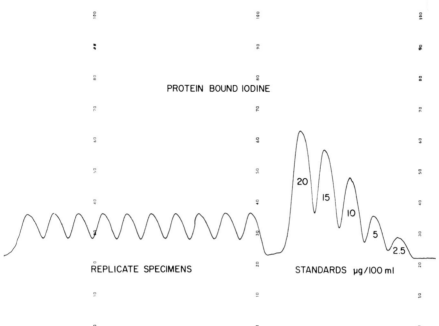

Fig. VIII-5.—Recorder tracing for total organic iodine.

13. After last sample has been recorded, turn heat off on digestor and remove Helix cover.

14. Turn off recorder.

15. Remove reagent lines from output manifold #2 and place in water.

16. Continue pumping reagents from input manifold #1 for 10 to 15 minutes while digestor is cooling.

17. Put reagent lines from input manifold #1 in water, continue pumping for 15 minutes to wash system out.

18. Turn off colorimeter.

Open proportioning pumps and relax end blocks.

Turn off digestor pump.

Turn off aspirator.

Calculations

The results are read directly from the chart recordings.

Precautions

High-quality reagents must be used throughout. On one occasion we obtained arsenous acid that was not usable. We found that it had been prepared from an inferior grade of arsenic trioxide. This lot resulted in unsatisfactory recorder patterns which were very irregular in contour.

A break in the acidflex tubing on the sample or waste pipet at the exit end of the digestor can cause excessive air bubbling and result in poor recordings. Routine inspection and maintenance should prevent this. After periodically replacing tubing on the manifolds (acidflex tubes each month), it is necessary to have three or four "runs" before the tubing is thoroughly softened and can produce good "peaks."

Inadvertent aspiration of a contaminated specimen into the regular, not contamination check, run may result in such gross contamination that all parts of the system in contact with the sample may have to be replaced. This may include the expensive digesting helix.

Difficulty may be encountered with the use of some commercially available control serums. There is unacceptable variation in the total serum organic iodine in some, an occasional lot having organic iodine levels of twice the stated values. It must be pointed out again that the method described measures total serum organic iodine rather than protein-bound iodine, and the relationship between these two values is not completely known. Better control serum is obtained by pooling a large number human sera and using aliquots as control serums over a many months' period. The reproducibility of our serum pool is $\pm 0.11 \ \mu g/100$ ml.

2. *Resin Nonextractable Iodine* ("Butanol Extractable Iodine," BEI)

Clinical Annotation

There are three conditions in which the measurement of total organic iodine or PBI does not provide a valid index of effective thyroid hormone levels. One is iodine overloading of the patient's serum with roentgenographic contrast media or ingestion of inorganic iodide compounds. At the present time, there are no chemical techniques which allow for the measurement of hormonal iodine in the presence of gross contaminating amounts of roentgenographic contrast media or ingested inorganic iodide substances. The second occurs in the patient with thyroiditis who produces large amounts of abnormal iodinated compounds which are physiologically inactive. The third occurs in some patients who have an inherited defect in thyroid biosynthesis.

Collection Notes

Blood collection is like that for total organic iodine.

Interpretation of Results

Hormonal iodine (thyroxine, butanol extractable iodine, or resin nonextractable iodine) usually accounts for 60 to 80 per cent of the total serum organic iodine or PBI. As the normal total serum organic iodine levels for the automated procedure (3.5 to 9.6 $\mu g/100$ ml.) are slightly higher, the normal levels for hormonal iodine are also slightly higher. Normal serum levels for our resin nonextractable iodine method range from 2.8 to 7.6 $\mu g/100$ ml.

Levels below 2.8 $\mu g/100$ ml. indicate hypothyroidism; conversely, elevated levels indicate hyperthyroidism.

Integrity of results depend on processing the sample and performance of the test with care. As with the total organic iodine method, the resin nonextractable iodine method described is vulnerable to impurities in alkaline reagents and to iodine, chlorine, and heavy metals in water used throughout the procedure.

METHOD

Principle

Quantitative butanol extraction of serum iodine consists of extraction procedures with n-butanol, subsequent treatments with alkaline reagents, and evaporation measures. In extraction, transfer and evaporation there are numerous chances for technical errors and iodine contamination. Moreover, the process is tedious and time consuming.

Ion exchange resins are useful in extracting inorganic iodine from serum specimens prior to analysis for organic iodine. With certain anion exchange resins columns, the process of removal of inorganic iodine may be very efficient and include some organic nonthyroid hormone iodine. Thus extraction of serum with these resins columns may replace butanol extraction. Our investigations show that one passage of 3 to 4 ml. of serum through a 3 cm. anion resin* column removes 98 per cent of added inorganic iodide. Added amounts up to 100 $\mu g/$ 100 ml. of serum are removed. Conversely, only 2 per cent of triiodothyronine and essentially no thyroxine is removed in the same procedure. Moreover, the values obtained correspond to those obtained with n-butanol extracted sera.

Preparation of Specimens and Resin Columns

Collect blood in iodine-free glassware† and separate serum. Prepare resin column by removing the cap and expressing the excess fluid. Tightly wind the closed end about a straight surgical clamp to express the last drops of fluid. Open the sealed end by cutting. Replace the small cap on the outlet of the column. Insert the outlet of the prepared column into the calibrated test tube supplied with the kit.

Resin Column Extraction Procedure

First, $3\frac{1}{2}$ ml. of serum are poured onto the column and allowed to stand for about 10 minutes. After this time, remove the cap to allow the column to drain. After the flow has spontaneously stopped, reapply the clamp and compress the column until exactly $3\frac{1}{2}$ ml. of serum has been expressed.

Analysis

The effluent serum is then analyzed for iodine, using the automated technique described for total organic iodine. The same aqueous iodate standards are used for both total organic iodine(PBI) and resin nonextractable iodine (BEI).

3. "T_3" Test (Estimation of Free Triiodothyronine)

Clinical Annotation

A relatively new index for thyroid function is the T_3 test. There are a large number of modifications of the original T_3 erythrocyte uptake procedure, but most are based upon the fact that thyroid binding proteins (TBP) bind most

---

*Rezikit, Squibb Medotopes, New Brunswick, N. J.

†Vacutainer tubes, Becton Dickinson.

Table VIII-7.—Selected Parathyroid Functional Disorders in Children

Disorder	Serum Calcium	Urine Calcium	Serum Inorganic Phosphate	Alkaline Phosphatase	Response to Parathormone
Idiopathic hypoparathyroidism	↓	↓	↑	N	N
Pseudo hypoparathyroidism	↓	↓	↑	N	0
Pseudo-pseudohypoparathyroidism	N		N	N	0
Primary hyperparathyroidism	↑	↑	↓	—	N
Secondary hyperparathyroidism (deficiency rickets, chronic renal failure, intestinal malabsorption)	↑	↓	↓	↑	N
Neonatal tetany	↓	—	↑	N	N
Vitamin D-intoxication	↑	N, ↑	N	N	N
Idiopathic infantile hypercalcemia	↑	—	N	N	N

of the circulating thyroid hormones (T_3 and T_4). The free, unbound hormone is metabolically active; hence, its measurement may more closely correlate with thyroid function than other measurements.

Moreover, this procedure usually is not invalidated by contaminating iodine, either ingested inorganics or roentgenographic contrast medias. Thus, it is a valuable test for patient seras with exogenous iodine contamination and as a measure of thyroid function in patients whose biologic fluids are temporarily overloaded with exogenous iodine.

Collection Notes

One milliliter of serum is used. Syringe and glassware precautions as for total organic iodine are exercised. No special preparation of the patient is necessary. Except in a few rare instances, neither organic nor inorganic exogenous iodide contamination interferes with the test.

Interpretation of Results

Circulating thyroid hormone is, for the most part, bound to specific plasma proteins, thyroid binding proteins. A small fraction, which is in equilibrium with the bound portion, circulates as a free thyroid hormone. The amount of free hormone determines the thyrometabolic status of the patient. In hyperthyroidism there is an increase, relative as well as absolute, in the amount of free thyroid hormones. The converse is true in hypothyroidism. When the plasma proteins are normal unbound T_3 mixed in serum ranges between 25 and 35 per cent of the added ^{131}I-L-triiodothyronine. Since the test is basically a measure of the binding power of the plasma proteins for L-triiodothyronine, alterations in the thyroid-binding fractions will also affect the results. Increases in thyroid-binding fractions occur in pregnancy, during estrogen treatment, in association with hydatidiform mole, sometimes with hepatitis and hepatic cirrhosis, and in instances of genetic alterations in the thyroid-binding protein fractions. Decreases in thyroid-binding fractions occur in nephrosis, exudative enteropathy, treatment with androgens, and in instances of genetic alterations of these thyroid-binding fractions. The free T_3 portion is reciprocally proportional to the concentrations of the thyroid-binding protein fractions.

METHOD

Principle

The serum specimen is mixed with tracer amounts of radioactive triiodothyronine. This trace amount of labeled exogenous hormone forms a homogenous mixture with the already present naturally occurring hormone. A count of total radioactivity is made. This mixture is allowed to react with an anion resin, which absorbs the unbound triiodothyronine. After washing, resin radioactivity is assayed. The per cent of radioactivity present in the resin is a measure of unbound triiodothyronine. The radioactivity not absorbed by the resin is an index of triiodothyronine bound to plasma proteins.

Materials

Originally, this test was developed using erythrocytes "in vitro." It is now more convenient to use one of the commercially available resin preparations of "sponges" which provide comparable data:

Manufacturer	Trade Name	Radioactive Label
Abbott	Triosorb	^{131}I
Squibb	Tresitope	^{125}I

Procedure

Complete and specific instructions are packaged with the commercial preparations and should be followed explicitly.

REFERENCES

ACTH RESERVE

1. Liddle, G. W., Estep, H. L., Kendall, J. W., Williams, C., and Townes, A. W.: Clinical application of a new test of pituitary reserve. J. Clin. Endocr. 19:875–890, 1959.

2. Steiker, D. D., Bongiovanni, A. M., Eberlein, W. R., and Leboeuf, G.: Adrenocortical and adrenocorticotropic function in children. J. Pediat. 59:884–889, 1961.

TSH RESERVE

1. Bishopric, G. A., Garrett, N. H., Nicholson, W. M.: Clinical value of the TSH test in diagnosis of thyroid diseases. Amer. J. Med. 18:15–19, 1955.

2. Bowers, C. Y., Morison, P. J., Gordon, D. L., and Locke, W.: Effect of thyrotropin on the serum protein-bound iodine level in various thyroid states (TSH-PBI test). J. Clin. Endocr. 2:465–471, 1961.

3. Jeffries, W. M., Levy, R. P., and Storaasli, J. P.: Use of the TSH test in the diagnosis of thyroid disorders. Radiology. 73:341–344, 1959.

4. Lamberg, B. A., Wahlberg, P., and Forsive, P. I.: The thyrotropin test in man using serum protein-bound iodine as an indicator. Acta Med. Scand. 153:411–420, 1956.

5. Pickering, D. E., and Miller, E. R.: Thyrotropic hormone in infants, and children; Differentiation between primary and hypopituitary hypothyroidism. Amer. J. Dis. Child. 85:135–140, 1953.

ADH RESERVE

1. Tests for diabetes insipidus. In Forsham, P. F. (Ed.): Endocrine System and Selected Metabolic diseases. Cibia Coll. Med. Illustr. vol. 4 by F. B. Netter, New York, Ciba, 1965, pp. 34–35.

2. Hsia, D. Y.-Y.: Nephrogenic diabetes insipidus. In Inborn Errors of Metabolism, ed. 2, part I: Clinical Aspects. Chicago, Year Book Publishers, 1966, pp. 278–380.

ADRENAL CORTEX RESERVE

1. DeFilippis, V., and Young, I. I.: Evaluation of adrenocortical function with intramuscular injection of ACTH gel. New Eng. J. Med. 257:1–6, 1957.

2. Ely, R. S., Raile, R. B., Bray, P. F., and Kelley, V. C.: Studies of 17-hydroxycorticosteroid; evaluation of a standard ACTH-17-hydroxycorticosteroid response test in children. Pediatrics. 13:403–411, 1954.

3. Jenkins, D., Forsham, P. H., Laidlaw, J. C., Reddy, W. J., and Thorn, C. W.: Use of ACTH in the diagnosis of adrenal cortical insufficiency. Amer. J. Med. 18:3–14, 1955.

4. Martin, M. M., and Wilkins, L.: Pituitary dwarfism; Diagnosis and treatment. J. Clin. Endocr. 18:679–693, 1958.

5. Soffer, L. J., and Gabrilove, J. L.: Simplified water loading test for the diagnosis of Addison's disease. Metabolism. 1:504–510, 1952.

6. Stone, D. B., and Jewel, J. G.: The danger of corticotropin in Addison's Disease. Arch. Intern. Med. 107:372–374, 1961.

CATECHOLAMINES AND VMA

1. Voorhess, M. L.: Urinary catecholamine excretion by healthy children. 1. Daily excretion of dopamine, norepinephrine, epinephrine and 3-methoxy-4-hydroxymandelic acid. Pediatrics 39:252–257, 1967.

2. Voorhees, M. L., and Gardner, L. I.: Studies of catecholamine excretion by children with neural tumors. J. Clin. Endocr. 22:126–133, 1962.

TOTAL ORGANIC IODINE

1. Austin, E., and Koepke, J. A.: An automated procedure for total organic iodine. Amer. J. Clin. Path. 45:344–347, 1966.

2. Chaney, A. L.: Protein-bound idoine. In Sobatka, H., and Stewart, C. P.: Advances in Clinical Chemistry, vol. 1. New York, Academic Press, Inc., 1958, pp. 82–109.

3. Oddie, T. H., and Fisher, D. A.: Protein-bound iodine levels during childhood and adolescence. J. Clin. Endocr. 27:89–92, 1967.

4. Riley, M., and Gochman, N.: A fully automated method for the determination of serum protein-bound iodine. Technicon International Symposium, New York, 1964.

5. Sunderman, F. W., and Sunderman, F. W., Jr.: The clinical significance of measurements of protein bound iodine. Amer. J. Clin. Path. 24:885–902, 1954.

BEI

1. Durham, J. R., Cook, R. E., Lancaster, J. W., and Mann, E. B.: Serum butanol-extractable iodine values of children under 10 years. Amer. J. Dis. Child. 87:468–474, 1954.

2. Man, E. B., and Bondy, P. K.: Clinical significance of serum butanol-extractable iodine J. Clin. Endocr. 17:1373–1382, 1957.

3. Man, E. B., Kydd, D. M., and Peters, J. P.: Butanol-extractable iodine of serum. J. Clin. Invest. 30:531–538, 1951.

4. Man, E. B., Pickering, D. E., Walker, J., and Cooke, R. E.: Butanol-extractable iodine in the serum of infants. Pediatrics. 9:32–37, 1952.

5. Taurog, A., and Chaikoff, I. L.: The nature of the circulating thyroid hormone. J. Biol. Chem. 176:639–656, 1948.

T_3 TEST

1. Crigler, J. F., Hertz, J., and Hamolsky, M. W.: In vitro red blood cell uptake of ^{131}I-L-triiodothyronine as a measurement of thyroid function in children. Amer. J. Dis. Child. 98:665, 1959.

2. Hamolsky, M. W., Godolitz, A., and Freedberg, A. S.: The plasma protein-thyroid hormone complex in man. III. Further studies on the use of the in-vitro red blood cell uptake of ^{131}I-L-triiodothyronine as a diagnostic test of thyroid function. J. Clin. Endocr. 19:103–116, 1959.

3. Hamolsky, M. W., Stein, M., and Freedberg, A. S.: The thyroid hormone-plasma protein complex in man. II. A new in vitro method for study of "uptake" of labelled hormonal components of human erythrocytes. J. Clin. Endocr. 17:33–44, 1957.

4. Koepke, J. A.: Correlation of bound T_3 with thyroid function. First Midwest Conference on the Thyroid. I:6, 1965.

5. Mitchell, M. L., Harden, A. B., and O'Rourke, M. E.: The in vitro resin-sponge uptake of triiodothyronine ^{131}I from serum in thyroid disease and pregnancy. J. Clin. Endocr. 20:1474–1483, 1960.

6. Nava, M., and DeGrot, L. J.: Resin uptake of I[131] labeled tri-iodothyronine as a test of thyroid function. New Eng. J. Med. 266:1307–1310, 1962.

CHAPTER IX

Aminoaciduria

Clinical Annotation

THE TWENTY MAJOR amino acids in blood range in individual concentrations between 1 and 4 mg. per cent. Thirty to forty appear in the urine, but only seven to nine account for 85 to 90 per cent of the total. Although there is much individual variation in the excretion of each amino acid, the excesses in pathologic aminoacidurias are easily recognized. An excess of individual or all amino acids may be ten to twenty times normal. The well described aminoacidurias are classified as shown.

Table IX-1.—Aminoacidurias

Disorder	Amino Acids/Metabolites in Excess	Pertinent Clinical Findings
I. *Aminoacidurias concerned with intermediary metabolism*		
A. *Hereditary*		
Overflow: Plasma concentration of one or more amino acid increased with consequent "overflow" into urine		
1. Citrullinemia	citrulline	mental retardation, vomiting, ammonia intoxication
2. Congenital lysine intolerance	lysine, arginine	periodic ammonia intoxication, spasticity
3. Histidinemia	histidine imidazolepyruvic acid $(FeCl_3 +)$ imidazolelactic acid imidazoleacetic acid	speech defect in many, mental retardation in many
4. Hyperglycinemia I	glycine	neonate: episodic vomiting, acidosis, ketosis later: seizures, mental retardation, neurologic deficits, neutropenia, thrombocytopenia; hypogammoglobinemia
5. Hyperglycinemia II	glycine with hypo-oxaluria	similar to type I without neutropenia and thrombocytopenia
6. Hyperlysinemia	lysine	hypotonia and lax ligaments, sparse hair, seizures, mental retardation
7. Hyperprolinemia I	proline, hydroxyproline, glycine	renal hypoplasia and disease, photogentic epilepsy, deafness, mental retardation
8. Hyperprolinemia II	proline; Δ'—pyrroline-5-carboxylic acid	mental retardation and convulsions

158

9. Hypervalinemia	valine	failure to thrive, vomiting, nystagmus
10. Hydroxy-prolinemia	hydroxyproline	mental retardation, microscopic hematuria
11. Maple syrup urine disease I	valine, leucine, isoleucine; plus respective keto acids (2,4 DPH +)	lethargy, anorexia, alternating hypertonicity and flaccidity with coma spasticity, seizures, mental retardation, usually early death
12. Maple syrup urine disease II	intermittent branch chained aminoaciduria and ketonuria as in Type I	symptoms as in Type I inter-mittant, may cause death
13. Methioninemia	methionine; others also in excess, α-keto-γ-methiol-butyric acid	progressive drowsiness, charac-teristic odor, cirrhosis, islet cell hyperplasia, renal tubular de-generation and early death
14. Oasthouse disease	phenylalanine, methio-nine, valine, leucine, isol-cucine and tyrosine; hydroxybutyric acid ($FeCl_3$ +)	mental retardation, white hair, edema, frequent infections, con-vulsions, abnormal odor
15. Hyper-ammonemia (Ornithine trans-carbamylase and carbamylphos-phate synthetase deficiencies)	compensatory increase in glutamine	chronic ammonia intoxication with vomiting, agitation and later stupor, mental retardation
16. Phenylketonuria, classical	phenylalanine, phenyl-pyruvic acid ($FeCl_3$ +) o-hydroxyphenylacetic acid	fairness of hair and skin, lethargy early, agitated behavior later, convulsions, eczema, and mental retardation
17. Phenylketonuria, atypical (several varieties due to separate defects)	phenylalanine, other metabolites variable	Patient seems normal, transient inactivity or immaturity of phenylalanine biodegradative enzymes in liver
18. Sarcosinemia	sarcosine	mental retardation
19. "T" substance anomaly	T-substance (ninhydrin reactive)	physical and mental retardation
20. Tyrosinosis	tyrosine p-hydroxyphenylpyruvic acid p-hydroxyphenyllactic acid p-hydroxyphenylacetic acid	cirrhosis of the liver, multiple renal tubular defects, vitamin D-resistant rickets, abnormal renal loss of water, hypokalemia, acidosis

No-Threshold: Amino acids concentrations in blood normal, large amounts are excreted in urine.

1. Argininosuccinic aciduria	argininosuccinic acid	ammonia intoxication, seizures, abnormal hair, mental retarda-tion
2. β-aminoiso-butyric aciduria	β-aminoisobutyric acid	benign, characteristic of Oriental population

3. Cystathionuria	cystathionine	mental retardation in some
4. Histidine peptiduria	carnosine, anserine, homo-carnosine methylhistidine	cerebromacular degeneration
5. Homocystinuria	homocystine	thromboembolic phenomena, ectopia lentis, osteoporosis, and sometimes mental retardation
6. Hypophospha-tasia	phosphoethanolamine	rickets-like bone disease, absence to trace serum alkaline phosphatase

B. *Acquired or transient*

1. Liver disease, all causes	generalized, especially tyrosine	——
2. Prematurity	generalized, especially proline and tyrosine	——
3. Steroid induced	generalized	——

II. *Aminoacidurias concerned with transport*

A. *Hereditary (primary)*

Amino acid concentrations in blood normal, large amounts are excreted in urine since renal tubular reabsorption is defective.

1. Cystinuria I	cystine, lysine, arginine, ornithine	cystine stones, slight growth faiure; heterozygotes excrete normal amounts of cystine and dibasic amino acids; intestinal transport absent for all dibasic amino acids
2. Cystinuria II	cystine, lysine, arginine, ornithine	cystine stones, slight growth failure, heterozygotes excrete moderate excesses of cystine and lysine; intestinal transport present for cystine only
3. Cystinuria III	cystine, lysine, arginine, ornithine	cystine stones, slight growth failure, heterozygotes excrete moderate excesses of cystine and lysine; intestinal transport present for all dibasic amino acids
4. Glycinuria with urolithiasis	glycine	calcium oxalate renal stones
5. Gluco-glycinuria	glycine	benign
6. Hartnup disease	gross amino aciduria (glutamine, histidine, serine threonine, phenyl-alanine tyrosine, trypto-phan), indole derivatives	pellagra-like skin rash, fluctuat-ing cerebellar ataxia, sometimes mental retardation and neurotic symptoms
7. Hyperglycinuria with iminoacid-uria	proline, hydroxyproline, glycine	rickets, hypophosphatemia, sometimes benign
8. Lowe's syndrome	generalized aminoaciduria with prominent glutamine	buphthalmus, cataracts, mental and physical retardation, hypo-tonia, hypophosphatemic rickets, and other renal tubular defects

| 9. Joseph's syndrome | proline, hydroxyproline, glycine | convulsions |
| 10. Tryptophanuria | tryptophan | dwarfism, mental retardation, photosensitivity, gait disturbance, pellagra-like rash |

B. *Hereditary (secondary)*

Transport defect not present at birth, but develops as result of progressive impairment of renal tubules by storage or cellular infiltrative substances.

1. Baber's congenital cirrhosis	generalized aminoaciduria	congenital cirrhosis with variety of renal tubular defects
2. Cystinosis	generalized aminoaciduria with prominent prolinuria	vitamin D resistant rickets, glycosuria, phosphaturia, chronic acidosis, hypokalemia and growth failure, progressive crystalline cystine deposits in all organs
3. Fanconi syndrome	generalized aminoaciduria	osteomalacia with hypophosphatemia resistant to vitamin D, hypokalemia hypouricemia, glucosuria and chronic acidosis
4. Galactosemia	generalized aminoaciduria	progressive liver failure leading to death or cirrhosis, cataracts and mental retardation
5. Wilson's disease	generalized aminoaciduria	progressive copper storage throughout life, liver failure and cirrhosis, Kayser-Fleischer rings of the cornea, progressive neurologic deterioration related to extra-pyramidal motor system

C. *Acquired*

Most aminoacidurias are due to impairment of renal tubules either by interference with their resorptive capacities or by transient cellular destruction. These "gross" or generalized aminoacidurias may be induced by drugs, poisons, abnormal metabolites, nutritional deficiencies and other causes. Proteinuria and glycosuria frequently accompany this type of aminoaciduria.

Collection Precautions

Urine. Freshly voided urine is submitted for analysis; a twenty-four-hour urine is not necessary for "screening." If collection or storage is prolonged, the specimen may be preserved either by freezing or by adding thymol or toluene, the former being preferable. Frequently, unusually discolored urine is submitted for analysis. This is usually the result of ingestion of drugs, dyes, or foods. A partial list of drugs which discolor urine is shown in tabular form.

Blood. Serum or heparinized plasma is suitable; storage is by freezing.

Table IX-2.—Drugs That Color the Urine

Blue

Methylene blue

Brown to Black

Aniline dyes	Naphthalene	Quinine
Cascara	Naphthol	Resorcinol (resorcin)
Chlorinated hydrocarbons	Nitrites	Rhubarb
Hydroxyquinone	Phenol	Santonin
Melanin	Phenyl salicylate (salol)	Senna
Methocarbamol (Robaxin)	Pyrogallol	Thymol

Green (Blue Plus Yellow)

Anthraquinone	Eosins	Resorcinol (resorcin)
Arbutin	Methocarbamol (Robaxin)	Tetrahydronaphthalene
Bile pigments	Methylene blue	Thymol

Magenta to Purple

Fuchsin
Phenolphthalein

Orange to Orange Red

Phenylazopyridine (Pyridium)

Orange to Red Brown

Combinations of phenylazopyridine (Pyridium) and other drugs used as urinary antiseptics; many of the trade names begin with *azo*.
Santonin

Pink and Red to Red Brown

Aminopyrine	Cinchophen	Emodin (alkaline urine)
Anthraquinone and its dyes	Danthron (Dorbane) (pink	Eosins (red with green
Antipyrine (Pyrazoline)	to violet-alkaline urine)	fluorescence)
Chrysarobi (alkaline urine)	Diphenylhydantoin (Dilantin)	
Hematuria producers (mercuric	Phenolphthalein	Thiazolsufone
salts, irritants, etc.)	(alkaline urine)	(Promizole)
Hemolysis producers	Phensuximide (Milontin)	Urates (especially new-
Phenindione (Danilone,	Porphyrins	born infants and dur-
Hedulin, Indon)	Prochlorperazine (Compazine)	ing tumor lysis)
Phenolic metabolites	Santonin (alkaline urine)	
(glucoronides)		

Rust Yellow or Brownish

Chlorzoxazone (Paraflex)	Liver poisons (Jaundice)	Naphthalene
Danthron (Dorbane)	Alcohol	Neocinchophen
(acid urine)	Arsenicals	Nitrofurantoins
Heavy metals (bismuth, mercury)	Carbon tetrachloride	Pamaquine
	Chloral hydrate	Sulfonamides
	Chlorinated hydrocarbons	Tribromomethanol with
	Chlorobutanol	amylene hydrate
	Chloroform	
	Cincophen	

Yellow or Green

Carotene-containing foods	Riboflavin	Yeast concentrate
Methylene blue	Vitamin B complex	

Adapted from Shirkey, H. C.: Reactions to drugs. In Pediatric Therapy, ed. 2. St. Louis, C. V. Mosby, 1966, pp. 56.

RAPID TUBE TESTS

1. *Ferric Chloride Test and*
2. *2,4-Dinitrophenylhydrazine Test*
    Described in Chapter XII in the discussion of phenylpyruvic acid.
3. *Homogentistic Acid Test*

Principle

Rapid oxidation of homogentesic acid, the excess metabolite in alcaptonuria, results in a brown-black opaque color of the urine. An additional characteristic of homogentisic acid is that it will develop unexposed photographic or X-ray film. Reactions with other test reagents yield characteristic color changes as described below.

Reagents

1. *Sodium Hydroxide (2.5 N)*

    | Sodium hydroxide | 100 Gm. |
    | Distilled water, q.s. | 1000 ml. |

    Dissolve the sodium hydroxide in distilled water and dilute to 1 L. volume.

2. *Millon's Reagent*

    | Metallic mercury | 10 Gm. |
    | Nitric acid, fuming (sp. gr. 1.420) | 11 ml. |
    | Distilled water, q.s. | 22 ml. |

    Mix metallic mercury and nitric acid. Dilute with distilled water. After a few hours, filter and store in a glass bottle.

3. *Ferric Chloride (10 Per Cent)*

    | $FeCl_3$ | 10 Gm. |
    | Distilled water, q.s. | 100 ml. |

    Dissolve the $FeCl_3$ in distilled water and store in dark bottle.

Procedure A and Interpretation

To 2 ml. of urine add 0.5 cc. of 2.5 N sodium hydroxide. Let stand for several minutes. The urine of an alkaptonuric individual turns a definite brown-black color on the addition of a strong oxidizing substance such as sodium hydroxide. A rapid additional confirmation test is to add a drop of urine and sodium hydroxide solution on to unexposed x-ray film. On photographic or x-ray film, alkaptonuric urine develops a dark spot on the film within 1 minute. Also, the Clinitest reaction for urine reducing substances ends in a "positive reaction."

Procedure B and Interpretation

Add Millon's reagent dropwise to the urine in a test tube. The appearance of a yellow precipitate turning red is a positive test for homogentisic acid.

Procedure C and Interpretation

Add Ferric chloride dropwise to the urine in a test tube. The appearance of a transient blue-violet color is a positive test for homogentesic acid.

4. *Cyanide-Nitroprusside Test*

Principle

Cyanide reduces cystine and homocystine to their thiol forms which then reacts with nitroprusside to give a purple color.

Reagents

1. *Ammonium Hydroxide (Concentrated)*

2. *Sodium Cyanide (Crystals)*

3. *Sodium Nitroferricyanide*

$NaFe(CN)_5(NO) \cdot 2H_2O$	5 Gm.
Distilled water, q.s.	100 ml

Store in refrigerator in opaque glass bottle.

Procedure and Interpretation

To 5 ml. of urine add 4 or 5 drops of concentrated NH_4OH and a few crystals of sodium cyanide. Mix and let stand 5 to 10 minutes. Add, dropwise, 5 per cent nitroprusside. A deep-purple color which fades gradually is a positive reaction. The intensity of the purple color is proportional to the concentration of either cystine or homocystine.

5. *Silver-Nitroprusside Test*

Principle

Silver nitrate, in the presence of excess sodium chloride, reduces homocystine to its thiol form. Cystine is not affected. Nitroprusside is added, then cyanide to give an immediate purple color. The specificity of the silver-nitroprusside test is based on the marked difference in reactivity of homocystine and cystine to the dismutative action of the silver diamine ion. Terminal addition of cyanide is required to bind the silver ion and permit reaction of homocystine with nitroprusside.

Reagents

1. *Sodium Chloride (Granular Form)*

2. *Ammonia*

Ammonium hydroxide, conc.	3 ml.
Distilled water, q.s.	100 ml.

Measure ammonium hydroxide into a 100 ml. volumetric flask and dilute to volume with distilled water.

3. *Silver Nitrate*

Silver nitrate	1 Gm.
Ammonia	100 ml.

Dissolve the silver nitrate in 100 ml. of ammonia.

4. *Sodium Nitroprusside*

NaFe $(CN)_5(NO) \cdot 2H_2O$	1 Gm.
Distilled water, q.s.	100 ml.

Dissolve the sodium nitroprusside in distilled water and dilute to a volume of 100 ml.

5. *Sodium Cyanide*

Sodium cyanide	700 mg.
Distilled water, q.s.	100 ml.

Dissolve sodium cyanide in distilled water and dilute to a volume of 100 ml.

Procedure and Interpretation

To 10 ml. of urine add sodium chloride (granular form) until saturated. Pipet 5 ml. of salt-saturated urine to a test tube. Add 0.5 ml. of silver nitrate solution. To a 5 ml. control sample of the salted urine add 0.5 ml. of ammonia (3 per cent). Let tubes stand 1 minute. To each tube add. 0.5 ml. of sodium nitroprusside and then 0.5 ml. of sodium cyanide. The development of an immediate pink to purple in the test sample *only* represents a positive test. The excess cyanide will begin to react with any cystine present to give a slowly forming positive cyanide-nitroprusside test.

6. *Millon Test*

Principle

The phenolic group of tyrosine and its derivatives react with mercuric ions to give a red-orange chelate.

Reagent

Millon's Reagent

Mercury, liquid metallic	10 Gm.
Nitric acid, fuming (sp. gr. 1.42)	11 ml.
Distilled water, q.s.	22 ml.

Dissolve the 10 Gm. of mercury in 11 ml. concentrated HNO_3, then dilute with 22 ml. of water. Let stand for several hours; filter and store in glass bottle.

Procedure and Interpretation

Apply 1 drop of urine to filter paper and allow to dry. Apply 1 drop of Millon's reagent and allow to dry. If tyrosine or p-hydroxy-phenylpyruvic acid is present in excess, an orange-brown ring will develop within 2 minutes. An alternate procedure is to add equal parts of urine and Millon's reagent in a test tube and heat to boiling. A red precipitate occurs if tyrosine or p-hydroxyphenyl-pyruvic acid is present in excess. Other derivatives of tyrosine (p-hydroxyphenyllactic acid, p-hydroxyphenylacetic acid and homogentesic acid) give a less intense positive reaction.

HIGH VOLTAGE PAPER ELECTROPHORESIS (HVPE)

Principle

HVPE is a method of partitioning closely related low molecular weight compounds. Electrically charged substances migrate in buffer on a filter paper support, the rate of migration of each substance depending upon their charge and degree of ionization. Classic chromatographic reagents are used to develop the partitioned substances. The intensity of the color development of the individual spots or bands is proportional to their concentrations.

Apparatus

A high-voltage electrophoresis system is manufactured by Savant Instruments, Inc., Hicksville, New York. Either the LT 36 or LT 22 tank may be used according to the width of the paper. Model HV 5000/3 high-voltage power supply is used. Mineral spirits* is the inert cooling material in direct contact with the support papers (see Figure Intro-9). An inexpensive cooling apparatus can be adapted from a drinking fountain refrigeration unit. We use model I-W-10A Kelvinator refrigeration unit manufactured by Kelvinator Water Cooler, Columbus, Ohio.

Preparation of Reagents

A. *Buffers with Electrophoretic Instructions*

1. *Buffer System: pH 2.0*

Formic acid	6 parts
Acetic acid, glacial	24 parts
Distilled water	170 parts

Operating voltage 1800 volts with potential gradient 20 v/cm.; current 80–85 ma; temperature 8 to 10°C; time 90 minutes.

2. *Buffer System: pH 3.6*

Pyridine	1 part
Acetic acid, glacial	10 parts
Distilled water	89 parts

Operating voltage of 1500 volts with potential gradient 30–35 v/cm.; current 85–90 ma; temperature 8 to 10° C.; time 30 minutes.

B. *Location Reagents with Development Instructions*

1. *Ninhydrin Stock*

Ninhydrin (Fisher certified or equivalent)	1.5 Gm.
Ethanol, 100 per cent	100.0 ml.

Store in dark bottle in refrigerator.

---

*Varsol, by Standard Oil of Kentucky.

2. *Ninhydrin Working Solution*

Ninhydrin stock	12 ml.
Chloroform	100 ml.
Pyridine	1 ml.

Mix just before use.

3. *Acid Copper Nitrate Solution*

Cupric nitrate, saturated soln.	1.0 ml.
HNO_3, 10 per cent	0.2 ml.
Ethanol, 100 per cent	99.0 ml.

Dip paper through the ninhydrin solution and allow to evaporate to dryness at room temperature. Place the paper in a vented chromatography oven for 20 minutes at 90° C. Maintain the environmental air (outside oven) at a relative humidity between 20 and 30 per cent. Then dip the paper through the acid copper nitrate solution and hang in an exhaust hood to dry. At this point, the rose-colored amino acid spots are stable for several months.

4. *Isatin*

Isatin	200 mg.
Acetone	98 ml.
Pyridine	2 ml.

Dip paper through the isatin solution and place in vented chromatography oven immediately. Allow development to continue for 10 minutes at 60° C. The amino acids develop various shades of blue on a yellow background. Proline, phenylalanine, and tyrosine stain most intensely, and are a characteristic robin's-egg-blue color.

5. *Alpha-nitroso-beta-naphthol:*

α-nitroso-β-naphthol	100 mg.
Acetone	20 ml.
Ethanol, 100 per cent	80 ml.

Dip paper through reagent and allow to dry at room temperature; redip through dilute HNO_3 (1 ml. conc. HNO_3 in 100 ml. 70 per cent ethanol) and allow to dry. Heat for 3 to 4 minutes at 90° C. Tyrosine gives a rose-colored spot on a light green background that begins to fade in 15 minutes.

6. *Sakaguchi Reagent*

a. *α-Naphthol Reagent*

α-Naphthol	100 mg.
Sodium hydroxide, 3N to 80 per cent ethanol	100 ml.

b. *N-Bromosuccinimide Reagent*

N-bromosuccinimide	1 Gm.
Acetone	100 ml.

The N-bromosuccinimide solution is to become yellow prior to using, usually requiring three to four hours. Dip paper through α-naphthol reagent and permit to dry partially at room temperature. Redip through N-bromosuccinimide reagent and again allow to dry at room temperature. The resulting pink band of arginine is stable for several days.

7. *p-Anisidine-amyl Nitrate*

p-Anisidine-amyl nitrate	1 Gm.
Ethanolic 0.1 N HCl	100 ml.
Amyl nitrite, 10 per cent in ethanol	100 ml.

Make fresh and allow to stand for 10 minutes. Dip paper through reagent and allow to dry at room termperature. Redip paper through ethanolic KOH. Histidine develops immediately at room temperature as a rose-colored spot on a light tan background; the color is stable for several hours.

C. *Standards*

The migrations of the individual amino acids from the separate origin spots are compared with the migrations of pure amino acids alone or added to urine. The distance traveled by each amino acid is compared to that of alanine (Mala), which is indicated by the number 1.00. Amino acid standards may be prepared individually or in the same solution.

1. *Stock Standards of Amino Acids.* Dissolve 1 millimole of each in 50 ml. water using a volumetric flask. Tyrosine, cystine and phenylalanine are less soluble and require larger volumes of water.

2. *Working Standards of Amino Acids.* Dilute 1 ml. of stock standard to 25 or 50 ml. in a volumetric flask. If diluted to 25 ml., 50 μL. contains 40 milli-micromoles (mμ moles). If diluted to 50 ml., 50 μL. contains 20 mμ moles.

Procedure

Preparation of Paper. Use large sheets (18¼ × 22½ in.) of Whatman No. 3 MM Chromatography paper. Mark the origin line 4 in. from, and parallel with, one of the 18¼ inch sides.

Preparation of Specimens

1. *Urine.* Apply directly to paper fifty microliters of unmodified urine at ¾ in. intervals along the "origin." In order to keep these spots about ¼ in. in diameter, make multiple applications of small aliquots of urine. For homocystine and cystine, best resolution can be obtained with prior oxidation to homocysteic and cysteic acids, respectively. Treat an aliquot of urine with an equal volume of freshly prepared performic acid solution (9 parts of 97 per cent formic acid and 1 part 30 per cent hydrogen peroxide, by volume). The oxidation of sulfhydryl and disulfide groups is complete within one hour. Pipet twice the usual (10 to 100 μL.) volume of urine onto the paper support.

2. *Plasma.* To 0.2 ml. plasma, add 1.0 ml. cold 95 per cent ethanol. Agitate

---

*Amino acids obtained either from Mann Research Laboratories, Inc., New York, N. Y., or from California Corporation for Biochemical Research, Los Angeles, California. Whenever possible, only chromatographically pure amino acids are used.

Table IX-3.—Amino Acid Migration Rates (pH 2.0)

Taurine	0.14	Leucine	0.78
Phosphoethanolamine	0.15	Isoleucine	0.79
Cystine (1/2)	0.55	Valine	0.83
Tryptophan	0.57	Serine	0.84
Tyrosine	0.60	Alanine	1.00
Hydroxyproline	0.61	Glycine	1.12
Aspartic acid	0.65	3-methylhistidine	1.25
Citrulline	0.65	Histidine	1.27
Phenylalanine	0.68	1-methylhistidine	1.27
Glutamic acid	0.71	β-aminobutyric acid	1.27
Glutamine	0.72	γ-aminobutyric acid	1.28
Methionine	0.72	β-alanine	1.39
Proline	0.75	Arginine	1.33
Asparagine	0.75	Lysine	1.41
Threonine	0.78	Ornithine	1.45

thoroughly, centrifuge at 300 × g. Apply 250 μL of supernatant in multiple small aliquots to the paper.

Electrophoresis

Choose a buffer which is best suited for the particular identification desired. Dip the paper through the buffer so that the entire paper is wet, except for ½ in. on either side of "origin" line. Mount the paper on the support rack and allow the dry area on either side of the origin line to become wet with buffer, either by capillary attraction or by spraying. Transfer the rack to the electrophoresis tank with the "origin" nearest the anode. Electrophorese the sample as specified under buffer preparation.

Cool the paper support by immersion in cold inert liquid (Varsol) which is kept cold by coils containing circulating water from a cooling unit.[*]

Color Development

Following electrophoresis, dry the papers at 90° C. for 20 minutes. Prepare the appropriate color developer and dip the paper through the solution; allow most of the location reagent to evaporate with the aid of a vigorous warm air blast for 30 to 60 seconds. Then, intensify the color development of the amino acids by heating. When a chromatography oven is used, it is vented and flushed with a stream of air (15 to 25 L./min.) which has a relative humidity of less than 15 per cent or compressed air that is forced through a gas drying cylinder[†] to the oven.

Identification

Primary identification of the amino acids is by their mobility. They are compared with known amino acids (standard solutions); secondary identification of the amino acids is by tints that are characteristic. Mobility rates (M_F) for amino acids using the pH 2.0 buffer are shown.

---

[*]Model IW-10A Kelvinator drinking fountain refrigeration units, manufactured by Kelvinator Water Coolers, Columbus, Ohio.

[†]Fisher No. 9–204 laboratory gas drying unit, a lucite cylinder packed with a moisture absorbing material, Drierite.

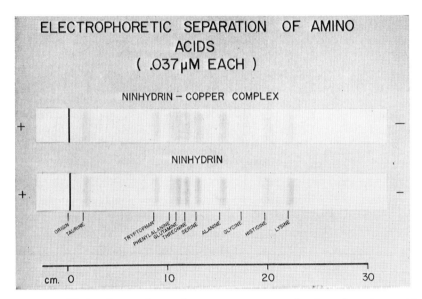

Fig. IX-1.—High-voltage electrophoretic separation of selected amino acids at 1500 v. × 90 min. Bands show the relative intensities of the ninhydrin and ninhydrin-copper development. The former location reagent fades over a period of days, the latter is permanent.

QUANTITATION OF INDIVIDUAL AMINO ACIDS

The individual amino acids and sugars are partitioned, developed, and identified as described in the preceding sections. Quantitation by means of comparisons with simultaneously run standards is desirable on occasion. To accomplish this, the standards and specimens must be applied as bands with a sample applicator.* They remain in bands during the electrophoretic partitioning. The papers are cut into strips 3 cm. in width and scanned with a recording densitometer-integrator.† Appropriate interference filters are used for the different colors:

500 mμ for pink bands
570 mμ for purple or lavender bands
600 mμ for blue bands

Scanning is facilitated by using neutral density filters to compensate for the background of the electrophoretic strips. The areas under the peaks are proportional to the color intensity and band widths; the integrator converts these peaks into units at the bottom of each tracing. The number of these units are proportional to the concentration of each amino acid in the specimen. Scanned strips are shown.

---

*No. 300–805 Spinco Division of Beckman Instruments, Inc., Palo Alto, Calif.

†Model R.B. Analytrol manufactured by Spinco Division of Beckman Instruments, Inc., Palo Alto, Calif. Optical density cam (B-2) used.

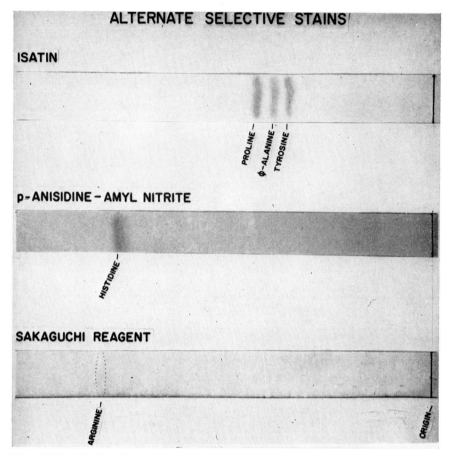

Fig. IX-2.—High-voltage electrophoretic separation of amino acids with selective development using special location reagents.

Quantities of individual amino acids are calculated as follows:

$$\frac{\text{integration units of unknown}}{\text{integration units of standard}} \times \frac{\text{quantity of standard on paper in m}\mu\text{ moles or }\mu\text{g}}{} \times \frac{\text{aliquot}}{\text{factor}} = \frac{\text{quantity of metabolite/}}{\text{unit volume}}$$

Normal values for individual urine and plasma amino acids, using these methods, are shown.

Interpretation of Results

Selected amino acid electrophoretograms in which the specimens were applied as bands at the origin are shown.

BETA-AMINOISOBUTYRIC ACID

Preparation of Reagents

A. *Buffer and Electrophoresis Instructions*

    1. *Buffer System, pH 3.6*

        Pyridine   1 part

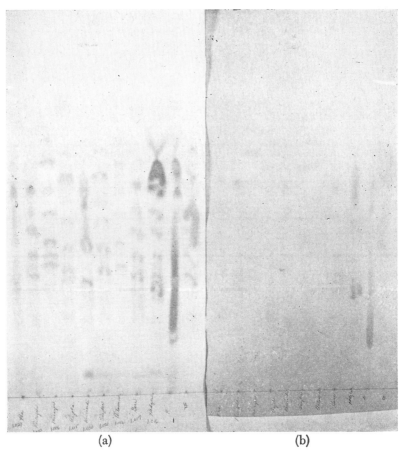

(a) (b)

Fig. IX-3.—"Screening" for pathologic aminoaciduria. Duplicate high-voltage electrophoretic separation of amino acids in 50 microliter aliquots of random urine from 11 patients (1500 v. × 90 min.). Electrophoretogram (a) developed with ninhydrin; (b) developed with isatin. Eight urines on left of each electrophoretogram normal. Three urines on right of each electrophoretogram are from patients with (9) cystinuria, (10) Fanconi syndrome, and (11) glycinemia. Specific gravity obtained on each specimen aids in estimation of amino acid concentrations. Trailing and smudging in pathologic specimens is due to overloading or large excesses of amino acid(s). Discrete patterns may be obtained with smaller volumes of urine.

Acetic acid, glacial	10 parts
Distilled water	89 parts

The operating potential is 20 volts/cm. length, current 4 to 5 ma per centimeter width; temperature at 10° to 15° C.; time 80 minutes. With our equipment, the voltage applied is 1 KV over 50 cm. length between buffer reservoirs.

B. *Location Reagent and Development Instructions*

1. Ninhydrin	200 mg.
2. Ethanol, 90 per cent	100 ml.

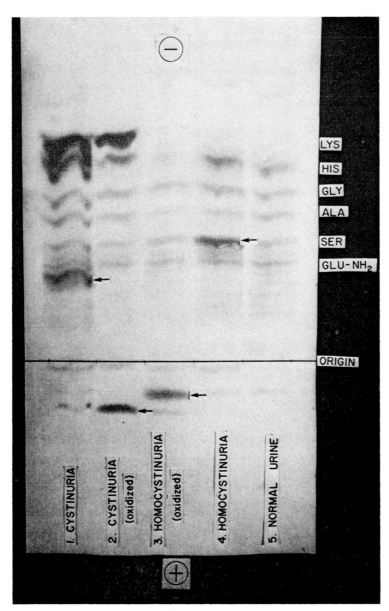

Fig. IX-4.—High-voltage electrophoretic separation of amino acids in urines from normal, homocystinuric and cystinuric patients. Prior oxidation of urine permits better resolution and identification.

Develop by dipping through ninhydrin solution and heating at 100° C. for 8 minutes.

Standard

Stock standard is prepared by dissolving 25 mg. BIBA in 250 ml. distilled

Table IX-4a.—Free Amino Acids in Normal Urine
(Micromoles per 24 Hours)

Amino Acid	Age Group					
	2 to 4 (11 Subjects)		4 to 6 (8 Subjects)		6 to 8 (12 Subjects)	
	Mean	Range	Mean	Range	Mean	Range
Lysine	54	24 to 89	54	17 to 148	59	27 to 159
Histidines	411	165 to 618	523	262 to 1,087	568	302 to 1,123
Glycine	399	175 to 693	599	395 to 1,008	467	166 to 723
Alanine	181	89 to 314	248	126 to 379	215	96 to 396
Serine	196	66 to 274	271	116 to 448	262	118 to 465
Glutamine	265	95 to 386	347	175 to 588	354	156 to 665
Taurine	178	42 to 299	223	89 to 399	214	42 to 467
Others	437	198 to 936	619	301 to 892	434	104 to 976
Total	2,121	1,229 to 3,133	2,884	1,537 to 4,225	2,573	

Table IX-4b.—Free Amino Acids in Normal Urine
(Micromoles per 24 Hours)

Amino Acid	(Years)							
	8 to 11 (12 Subjects)		11 to 15 (8 Subjects)		15 to 21 (7 Subjects)		21 to 35 (50 Subjects)	
	Mean	Range	Mean	Range	Mean	Range	Mean	Range
Lysine	101	28 to 396	88	28 to 188	114	76 to 160	245	31 to 852
Histidine	629	232 to 1,130	619	384 to 966	765	459 to 975	1,387	610 to 3,026
Glycine	672	302 to 1,436	838	421 to 1,631	955	316 to 1,224	1,272	692 to 2,196
Alanine	308	146 to 628	341	208 to 667	306	244 to 410	500	274 to 975
Serine	341	190 to 516	369	238 to 606	378	335 to 414	617	125 to 1,125
Glutamine	490	242 to 844	482	278 to 899	447	378 to 527	805	401 to 1,447
Taurine	349	24 to 895	255	60 to 391	200	182 to 527	593	141 to 1,277
Others	674	122 to 1,435	506	136 to 1,408	829	462 to 1,087	1,420	25 to 3,374
Total	3,537	1,412 to 6,059	3,498	2,246 to 6,221	4,094	3,504 to 4,423	6,839	3,516 to 11,812

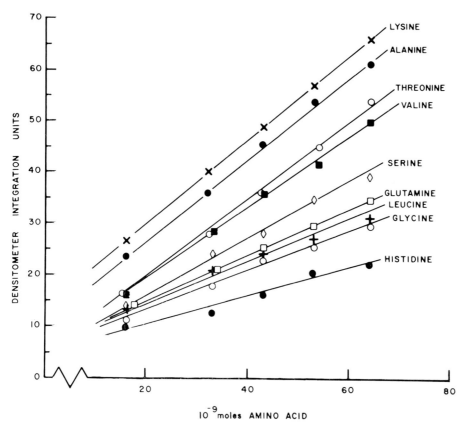

Fig. IX-5.—Representative amino acid proportionality data using ninhydrin-copper location reagent.

water using a volumetric flask. Standards applied to paper are

$$20 \, \mu L. = 2 \, \mu g$$
$$40 \, \mu L. = 4 \, \mu g$$
$$60 \, \mu L. = 6 \, \mu g$$

Procedure

Preparation of Paper. On Whatman No. 3 MM filter (22 by 57 cm.) paper, draw the "origin" line across the shorter dimension, 12 cm. from one end and apply the specimen as a spot or band and dry.

Electrophoresis. The paper is dampened with buffer, care being taken not to wet the area of spot application directly with the buffer, but rather to allow the buffer to diffuse slowly into this region. The sheet is then suspended on the support rack and placed in the electrophoresis tank.

Staining and Color Development. Upon removal from the tank, dry the paper at 90° C. in an air-vented chromatography oven for 20 minutes. Then, dip it through the location reagent and heat at 100° C. in the chromatography oven for 8 minutes.

Table IX-5.—Normal Plasma-free Amino Acids

Amino Acid(s)	12 Prematures μM/1	12 Newborns μM/1	12 Infants μM/1	12 Children μM/1	12 Young Adults μM/1	Published Values μM/1
Lysine	261‡ (144-376)*	234‡ (82-420)	212‡ (128-308)*	121‡ (69-174)*	117‡ (77-209)*	45-144
Histidine	171 (87-305)	135 (60-237)	191 (95-380)	128 (83-191)	147 (41-228)	24-112
Glycine	233 (160-337)	344 (253-457)	187 (67-320)	211 (84-353)	220 (137-311)	56-308
Alanine	280 (164-408)	320 (223-506)	320 (175-461)	214 (80-362)	296 (240-380)	99-313
Serine-valine	281 (176-379)	212 (127-332)	321 (202-561)	218 (106-320)	184 (135-219)	51-434
Leucine-threonine	254 (135-390)	181 (104-293)	262 (160-335)	147 (76-200)	172 (133-209)	78-283
Glutamic acid-glutamine	686 (571-900)	702 (381-956)	701 (465-965)	422 (236-662)	577 (428-818)	46-290
Proline	250 (117-351)	198 (105-335)	257 (123-369)	104 (63-166)	118 (70-208)	51-185
Phenylalanine	120	120	120	120	120	23-69

‡Mean.
*Range.

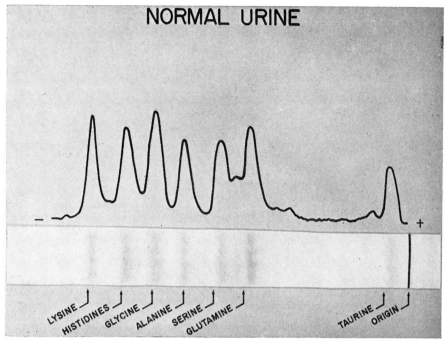

Fig. 1A-6.—High-voltage electrophoretogram of normal urine. Subsequent scanning with recording densitometer provides method for quantitation. Further separation of individual bands can be obtained by electrophoresing for a longer period of time.

Identification and Calculations. Identify the β-aminoisobutyric acid by its migration rate. The intensity of the spot or band of the specimen is compared with standards. Express the amount of BIBA excreted as mg./24 hr. An alternate method using an untimed, randomly voided, urine specimen is to determine the amount of BIBA in a volume of urine containing 1 Gm. of creatinine. This is practical, since creatinine excretion is relatively constant.

Sample Calculations

A. Ratio of unknown compared to standard × mg. standard on paper ×

$$\frac{\text{volume 24 hr. urine}}{\text{volume urine applied to paper}} = \text{mg. BIBA excreted/day}$$

B. Ratio of unknown compared to standard × mg. standard on paper ×

$$\frac{\text{vol. urine containing 1 Gm. creatine}}{\text{vol. urine applied to paper}} = \text{mg. BIBA/Gm. creatine excreted}$$

REFERENCES

1. Bessman, S. P., Koppanyi, Z. H., and Wapnir, R. A.: A rapid method for homocystine assay in physiological fluids. Anal. Biochem. 18:213–219, 1967.

2. Blumberg, B. S., and Gartler, S. M.: High prevalence of high-level β-amino-isobutyric acid excretors in micronesians. Nature (London). 184:1990–1992, 1959.

3. Efron, M. L., Young, D., Moser, H. W., and MacCready, R. A.: A simple chromatographic screening test for the detection of disorders of amino acid metabolism. New Eng. J. Med. 270:1378–1783, 1964.

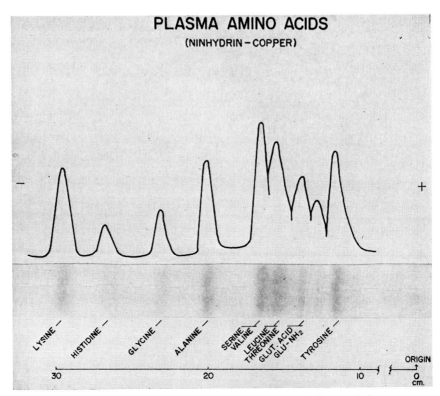

Fig. IX-7.—High-voltage electrophoretogram of normal plasma. Subsequent scanning with recording densitometer provides method for quantitation.

4. Gartler, S. M.: A metabolic investigation of urinary β-aminoisobutyric acid excretion in man. Arch. Biochem. 80:400–409, 1959.

5. Hsia, D. Y.: The screening of hereditary metabolic defects among newborn infants. Canad. Med. Assoc. J. 95:247–251, 1966.

6. Lewis, H. B.: Cystinuria; a review of some recent investigation. Yale J. Biol. Med. 4:437–449, 1931–1932.

7. Mabry, C. C., and Karam, E. A.: Measurement of free amino acids in plasma and serum by means of high-voltage paper electrophoresis. Amer. J. Clin. Path. 42:421–430, 1964.

8. Mabry, C. C., and Todd, W. R.: Quantitative measurement of individual and total free amino acids in urine; Rapid method employing high-voltage paper electrophoresis and direct densitometry and its application to the urinary excretions of amino acids in normal subjects. J. Lab. Clin. Med. 61:146–157, 1963.

9. Perry, T. L., Hansen, S., and MacDougall, L.: Urinary screening tests in the prevention of mental deficiency. Canad. Med. Assoc. J. 95:89–95, 1966.

10 Renuart, A. W.: Screening for inborn errors of metabolism associated with mental deficiency or neurologic disorders or both.New Eng.J.Med.274:384–387,1966.

11. Sackett, D.: Adaptation of monodirectional high-voltage electrophoresis on long papers to the rapid qualitative identification of urinary amino acids. J. Lab. Clin. Med. 63:306–314,1964.

12. Samuels, S.: High-resolution screening of amino-acidurias. Arch. Neurol. 10:322–326, 1964.

13. Spaeth, G. L., and Barber, G. W.: Prevalence of homocystinuria among the mentally retarded: Evaluation of a specific screening test. Pediatrics 40:586–589, 1967.

CHAPTER X

Glycosuria and Glycorrhea

Clinical Annotation

GLUCOSE ACCOUNTS FOR almost all carbohydrate in blood, although transient amounts of other sugars may appear following their ingestion. It follows that transient glucosuria is the only normal glycosuria that occurs to a measureable degree by copper reduction and that many dietary sugars appear in the urine in scanty, hardly measureable amounts. When defects in the intestinal hydrolysis and absorption of sugars are present, (1) the unhydrolyzed disaccharides that cross the intestinal barrier appear almost quantitatively in the urine and (2) gross amounts of the either unhydrolyzed or unabsorbed sugar(s) appear in the stool. When there is impairment of renal tubular reabsorption of sugars, the urine contains excesses of the respective sugar(s). The recognized glycosurias and glycorrheas may be classified as (1) hereditary or acquired, (2) according to major site of defect, and (3) by the individual sugar affected.

Table X-1.—Glycosurias and Glycorrheas

A. Hereditary Disorders

    I.   Glycosurias associated with defects in intermediary metabolism.

1. Diabetes mellitus	Manifestations those of deficiency of insulin. Time of onset and clinical severity varies greatly. Glucosuria follows hyperglucosemia.
2. Galactokinase deficiency	Juvenile cataracts. Galactokinase activity absent. Galactosuria follows hypergalactosemia.
3. Galactosemia	Persistent jaundice at birth with liver impairment. Develop cirrhosis, cataracts, mental retardation, seizures. Galactose-1-PO_4-uridyl transferase activity absent. Galactosuria follows hypergalactosemia. A less severe and genetically distinct form, with diminished enzyme activity, is the Duarte variety.
4. Benign fructosuria	No symptoms and harmless. Results from inability to metabolize fructose; defect unknown. Fructose accumulated in blood excreted in urine.
5. Fructose intolerance	Fructose induces hypoglycemia and toxic symptoms of vomiting, jaundice and hepatosplenomegaly, Fructose-1-PO_4-aldolase absent. Fructosuria related to fructosemia.
6. Lactose intolerance	Anorexia, vomiting, diarrhea with failure to thrive. Lactosemia and lactosuria without abnormal increase in glucose may be transient after first weeks of life.
7. Lipoatrophic diabetes	Persistent hyperglucosemia without ketosis. Accelerated growth, hepatomegaly and absence of all body fat. Defect not determined. Glucosuria dependent on hyperglucosemia.

Table X-1.—Continued

8.	Pentosuria	No symptoms — a harmless disorder. L-xylulosuria in great excess.
9.	Pseudo-phlorizin diabetes	Characterized by growth failure, hepatomegaly, transient periods of hyperglycemia but with persistent excessive glucosuria, mild ketosis, and diabetic glucose tolerance. Not insulin dependent.

II. Glycosurias associated with defects in renal tubular transport.

1.	Glucoglycinuria	A combined defect of transport of glycine and glucose. Normal blood levels of both glycine and glucose. No symptoms.
2.	Renal glycosuria	Defect limited to transport of glucose. Characterized by low renal threshold for glucose. No symptoms.
3.	Associated with other severe tubular defects (e.g. Fanconi syndrome, Cystinosis, Lowe's syndrome)	

III. Deficiency of intestinal sugar-splitting or absorbing enzymes.

1.	Sucrose-isomaltase deficiency	Diarrhea of variable intensity with abdominal distention and poor growth when sucrose fed. Sucrorrhea and iso-maltorrhea.
2.	Lactose deficiency	Diarrhea of variable intensity following lactose ingestion. Abdominal distension and poor growth when lactose fed. Lactosuria prominent feature as is lactorrhea. Stool pH low, and renal function may be disturbed.
3.	Glucose-galactose malabsorption	Diarrhea of variable intensity following lactose, glucose and galactose. Abdominal distension and poor growth when these sugars are fed. Glycosuria mild; galactorrhea and glucorrhea.

B. Secondary Disorders

    I. Glycosurias associated with defects in intermediary metabolism (glucosurias).
        1. Destruction of pancreatic islet cell tissue (e.g. surgical removal, pancreatitis, tumor, hemochromatosis)
        2. Acromegaly
        3. Adrenal hyperfunction
           a) Cortical
           b) Medullary
        4. Thyroid hyperfunction
        5. Carbohydrate challenge following starvation

    II. Glycosurias associated with defects in renal tubular transport; glucosurias

        These result from cellular damage as with mercury or lead poisoning or impaired function due to some drugs or chemicals.

    III. Deficiency of intestinal sugar-splitting or absorbing enzymes

        The disaccharide splitting enzymes are located in the brush border of the upper intestinal epithelium. Monosaccharide transport occurs in the epithelial cells. Thus, these enzymes and mechanisms may be impaired whenever ulcerative, inflammatory, granulomatous, atrophic, infiltrative, or other anatomic abnormalities are present. Thus disacchariduria and glycorrhea may occur with infectious diarrhea, celiac disease, cystic fibrosis, ulcerative colitis, regional enteritis, giardiasis, and other intestinal disorders. Lactulose, a derivative of lactose, has been observed in urine, usually with intestinal lactase deficiency.

Collection Notes

Freshly voided urine or passed stool is suitable for analysis. Liquid stool is collected by using a plastic urine bag. Specimens are tested as soon as possible or are frozen until the time of analysis. A timed or twenty-four hour urine or stool collection is rarely needed.

RAPID TUBE TESTS

1. Reducing Substances

Principle

Many normal excretory products are reducing substances; however, they do not usually occur in sufficient concentrations to be detected by a copper reduction test. The reduced copper, cuprous oxide, is readily detectable. As the number of cuprous oxide particles increases, the color of the precipitate varies from green to yellow to orange.

Reagents

1. *Benedict's Reagent*

Sodium carbonate, anhydrous	100.0 Gm.
Copper sulfate	17.3 Gm.
Sodium citrate	173.0 Gm.
Distilled water, q.s.	1000.0 ml.

Place sodium carbonate in about 100 ml. of distilled water. Add the sodium citrate and heat to dissolve. Allow to cool to room temperature. Dissolve the copper sulfate in about 100 ml. of water. Pour the copper sulfate solution slowly into the solution of carbonate and citrate salts. Make up to 1 L. with distilled water and mix.

Procedure

Use undiluted urine or an aqueous stool eluate. The stool eluate is prepared by (1) placing a small volume of stool in a centrifuge tube, (2) diluting to twice its volume with water, (3) mixing well, (4) centrifuging, and (5) using the cleared supernatant. Place about 7 drops of urine or 20 drops of stool supernatant into a test tube. Add 5 ml. of Benedict's reagent. Place the tube in a boiling water bath for 5 minutes. If reducing substances are present, they will reduce the copper in the Benedict's solution. The color will vary from green to yellow to orange depending upon the amount of reducing substances present.

For a quicker method, Ames Clinitest® tablets may be used. For urine, place 5 drops in a test tube and add 10 drops of water. For stool, add 15 drops of supernatant to a test tube without additional water. Add 1 tablet. Allow reaction to continue for about 1 minute or until there is no turbulence in the test tube. If reducing substances are present, the color reaction will vary from green to yellow to orange depending on concentrations of the reducing substances.

All sugars expected in urine or stool, except sucrose, are reduced under these conditions, but with varying intensities. If sucrose is thought to be present in a specimen, the sucrose may be hydrolyzed with dilute hydrochloric acid to its component monosaccharides, fructose and glucose. In actual experience with patients who have either congenital or acquired sucrose intolerance, they pass sufficient glucose and fructose in their stools to give a positive reducing reaction. This presumably results from the hydrolysis of sucrose by the intestinal flora before the stool is passed.

Results and Interpretations

The colors obtained indicate the concentration of sugar with the reducing capacity of glucose as follows:

Reaction Color	Approximate Concentration	Significance Urine	Stool
Blue	0	negative	negative
Green	¼ Gm.%	trace	negative
Olive	½ Gm.%	+	suspicious
Yellow-green	¾ Gm.%	+ +	abnormal
Yellow-brown	1 Gm.%	+ + +	abnormal
Orange	2 Gm.%	+ + + +	abnormal

2. Glucose Oxidase Reaction

Glucose may be specifically identified in urine by using paper strips* impregnated with glucose oxidase. Glucose oxidase reacts with glucose to remove two hydrogen ions, forming gluconolactone which is hydrated to gluconic acid. The removed hydrogen ion is then combined with atmospheric oxygen to form hydrogen peroxide.

The over-all reaction is expressed as follows:

$$glucose + O_2 \xrightarrow{glucose\ oxidase} gluconic\ acid + H_2O_2$$

The H_2O_2, in the presence of peroxidase, oxidizes orthotolidine which in its oxidized state turns blue.

$$H_2O_2 + orthotolidine \xrightarrow{peroxidase} oxidized\ orthotolidine\ (blue) + H_2O$$

The intensity of the blue color is proportional to the concentration of glucose in pure aqueous solutions. In biologic fluids such as urine, this is not always true. Vitamin C and the tetracyclines excreted in patients' urines inhibit glucose oxidase activity and give spuriously low or negative results. Timing the reaction (10 seconds) is essential, since in time the peroxidase reaction will go to completion and give a dark blue color.

HIGH VOLTAGE PAPER ELECTROPHORESIS (HVPE)

Principle

Sugars do not ionize alone in aqueous solution, but may do so when

*Tes-Tape by Eli Lilly and Company. Clinistix by Ames Co.

complexed with other radicals. Thus, usually electrically neutral sugars become charged substances in the presence of borate radicals. The individual sugars then move in an electrical field in buffer on paper, with the rate of migration of the individual sugars depending on their charge and degree of ionization. Partitioning is rapid and discrete. Classic chromatographic locating reagents are used to develop the partitioned sugars. The intensity of the color development of the individual spots or bands is proportional to their concentrations.

Apparatus

HVPE systems manufactured by Savant Instruments, Inc., Hicksville, New York are used in our laboratory. Either the LT 36 or LT 22 tank may be used according to the width of the paper. A Model HV 5000/3 power supply is used. Mineral spirits (Varsol) as marketed by Standard Oil of Kentucky is the inert cooling material in the electrophoresis tanks. Equipment distributed by other companies has been found suitable by others.

Preparation of Reagents

A. *Buffers with Electrophoretic Instructions*

    1. *Buffer System: pH 9.2*

Sodium borate	38.1 Gm.
Distilled water	1000.0 ml.

    The operating potential is 24 volts per centimeter length, current 4 to 5 ma/cm. width; temperature at 8 to 10° C.; time 150 minutes. With our equipment, the voltage applied is 1.2 KV over 50 cm. length between buffer reservoirs.

    2. *Buffer System: pH 6.3*

Boric acid	39.0 Gm.
Distilled water	1000.0 ml.

    Add 1M NaOH dropwise until the desired pH is obtained. The operating potential gradient is 40 V/cm. length, current 1 to 2 ma/cm. width, temperature 10 to 12° C.; time 120 minutes. With our equipment, the voltage applied is 2.0 KV over 50 cm. length between buffer reservoirs.

B. *Location Reagents with Development Instructions*

    1. a. Diphenylamine   2.0 mg.

a. Diphenylamine	2.0 mg.
Orthophosphoric acid	8.8 ml.
Acetone	100.0 ml.
b. p-Anisidine	2.0 mg.
Orthophosphoric acid	8.8 ml.
Ethanol, 100 per cent	100.0 ml.

    Combine equal parts of reagents a and b. The resulting mixture is filtered to remove excess phosphate. Papers are dipped through the filtered reagent, and acetone and ethanol are evaporated by drying at room temperature for 20 minutes. Papers are placed in a thermostatically controlled vented chromatography oven for 10 to 15 minutes

Table X-2.—Mobilities and Colors of Sugars

Sugar	M Glucose (pH 9.2)	M Ribose (pH 7.3)	Color (pH 9.2)
D-glucuronic acid	1.25	Streaked	Copper
D-galacturonic acid	1.16	1.56	Copper
D-glucose	1.00	Streaked	Green
D-xylose	1.00	Streaked	Green-gray
D-fucose	0.96	Streaked	Yellow
D-arabinose	0.95	Streaked	Copper
D-sorbose	0.95	1.27	Yellow-green
D-galactose	0.90	Streaked	Green
D-fructose	0.88	1.16	Gold
Melibiose	0.79	Streaked	Yellow-green
D-erythrose	0.78	Streaked	Gold
D-ribose	0.69	1.00	Yellow-green
D-xyulose	0.69	1.22	Gold
D-lyxose	0.68	0.54	Green-gray
D-mannose	0.68	0.31	Green
Turanose	0.61	0.38	Green-yellow
D-rhamnose	0.46	Streaked	Gold
Lactose	0.36	−0.08	Green
N-acetyl-D-galactosamine	0.30	−0.10	Green
Maltose	0.28	−0.15	Green
D-2-deoxyribose	0.27	−0.16	Copper
D-2-deoxyglucose	0.25	−0.23	Copper
Cellobiose	0.24	−0.25	Yellow-green
Raffinose	0.19	−0.19	Yellow-green
Stachyose	0.17	−0.13	Yellow-green
N-acetyl-D-glucosamine	0.13	−0.26	Green
Gentianose	0.09	−0.28	Yellow-green
Sucrose	0.09	−0.27	Tan
Inulin	0.07	−0.26	Yellow

at 85° C. with a relative humidity of 30 ± 5 per cent. The colors developed are listed.

2. *Diphenylamine-Aniline Reagent*

Diphenylamine	1.0 Gm.
Aniline	1.0 ml.
Acetone	100.0 ml.
Orthophosphoric acid, 85 per cent	15.0 ml.

The white precipitate disappears with mixing. Dip paper through reagent and allow to evaporate to near dryness at room temperature. Place paper in vented chromatography oven for 6 minutes at 90° C. with the relative humidity of 30 + 5 per cent.

3. *Aniline-Phthalate Reagent*

Aniline (aminobenzene)	1.0 ml.
Phthalic acid	1.7 Gm.
n-Butanol, water saturated	100.0 ml.

Dip paper through reagent and allow to dry at room temperature for 30 minutes. Place paper in vented chromatography oven at 100 to 105° C. for 10 minutes. All sugars are stained a uniform tan color.

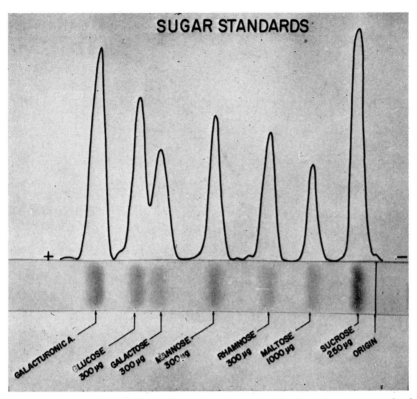

Fig. X-1.—High-voltage electrophoretic separation of selected sugar standards at 1200 volts for 120 minutes. Subsequent development and scanning with a recording densitometer provides method for quantitation.

Standards

Monosaccharides are dissolved in 10 per cent isopropanol as 500 mg. per cent solutions; oligosaccharides are prepared similarly as 1000 mg. per cent solutions. Two convenient mixtures of initial standards are used.

   a. glucose, fructose, mannose, lactose
   b. glucose, galactose, maltose, sucrose

Store in refrigerator. Usually 50 μL. of standard solution is applied at the origin; this is equivalent to 250 μg and 500 μg of monosaccharides and disaccharides, respectively.

Procedure

Preparation of Paper. Whatman No. 3 MM filter paper, 57 by 23.5 or 47 cm. is used; the origin line is drawn across the shorter dimension, 12 cm. from one end. The volume of the specimen applied varies according to the expected concentration of the sugars. Best resolution is obtained by using a sample applicator.* Usually 25 μL. of standard solution is applied to the origin; this is

---

*No. 300-805 Spinco Division of Beckman Instruments, Inc., Palo Alto, Calif.

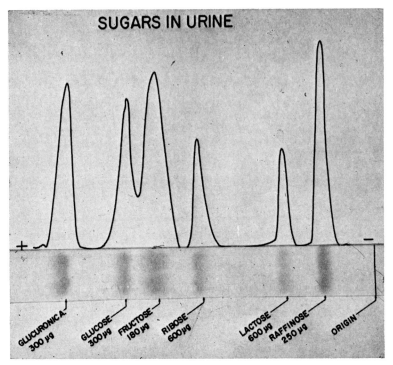

Fig. X-2.—High-voltage electrophoretic separation of multiple sugars added to urine at 1200 volts for 120 minutes. Subsequent development and scanning with a recording densitometer provides method for quantitation.

equivalent to 125 and 250 μg of monosaccharides and oligosaccharides, respectively.

Preparation of Specimens. An amount of sugar solution approximating 250 μg of sugar(s) is applied to the origin. These amounts are determined according to the Clinitest† reaction.

Color	Specimen Volume Applied	Color	Specimen Volume Applied
blue	100μL	yellow	25μL
green	50μL	orange	10μL

For specimens requiring extraction, larger volumes are applied. Ordinarily, protein-containing material such as serum does not have to be deproteinized, but ethanolic solutions are easier to apply even though more dilute. The techniques used are:

URINE: Applied directly to paper.

SERUM: One hundred to 200 μL. of serum is applied directly to paper; or, to 0.25 ml. of serum is added 1.0 ml. of 95 per cent ethanol, and the mixture is agitated and centrifuged at 1500 rpm for 10 minutes after which 500 μL. or more of supernatant is applied.

---

†Manufactured by Ames Company, Inc., Elkhart, Indiana.

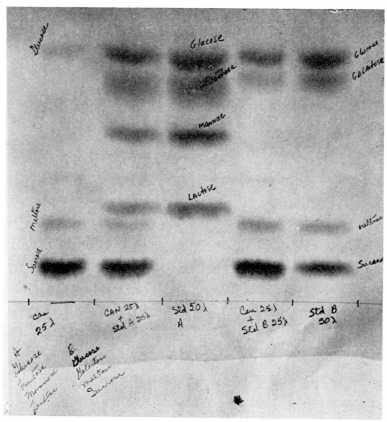

Fig. X-3.—High-voltage sugar electrophoretogram which shows how sugars in a newly marketed infant milk were identified. Left to right (1) new infant milk, (2) new infant milk with mixture of sugar standards, (3) mixture of sugar standards, (4) new infant milk with mixture of alternate sugar standards, and (5) mixture of alternate sugar standards.

STOOL: Approximately 2 ml. of 70 per cent ethanol is added to each gram of homogenized stool. After adequate mixing the specimen is centrifuged, and an aliquot of supernatant is applied.

ELECTROPHORESIS: The paper is dipped through the buffer until all but 1 to 2 cm. on either side of the origin has become saturated. The paper is placed on the rack support, and the remaining dry area is sprayed lightly with buffer. The rack is lowered into the electrophoresis tank containing buffer in the lower chambers and an inert solvent (Varsol) which serves as a cooling medium in the remainder. The electrophoresis chamber is cooled by continuously circulating a permanent antifreeze solution through a refrigeration unit and the coils of the chamber. The origin is placed near the negative (cathode) terminal.

STAINING AND COLOR DEVELOPMENT: After removal from the electrophoresis chamber, the papers are suspended and dried in a chromatography oven at 90° C. for 30 minutes. Papers are dipped through the location

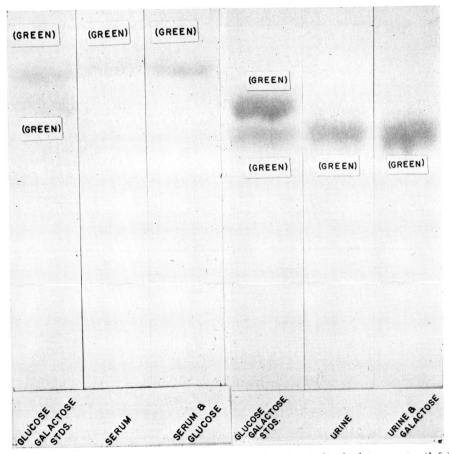

Fig. X-4.—High-voltage electrophoretograms showing individual sugars in (left) the serum of a prematurely born infant following a cow's milk feeding, and (right) the urine of a patient with galactosemia.

reagent selected, then dried at room temperature. Then the papers are placed in a thermostatically controlled, vented chromatography oven for a length of time (depending on the location reagent being used) at a relative humidity of 30 per cent. Intermittent observations may be made to note the rate of appearance of the characteristic colors of the individual bands.

IDENTIFICATION: The individual sugars are identified by three properties: mobility, color, and rate of color development. Mobility rates are determined by their relation to the mobility of glucose (M_G) at pH 9.2 and the mobility of ribose (M_R) at pH 7.3. These sugars are included among the standards in each run. The colors of the individual sugars develop at different rates, and the sugars have characteristic colors which aid in their identification. Selected electrophoretograms are shown.

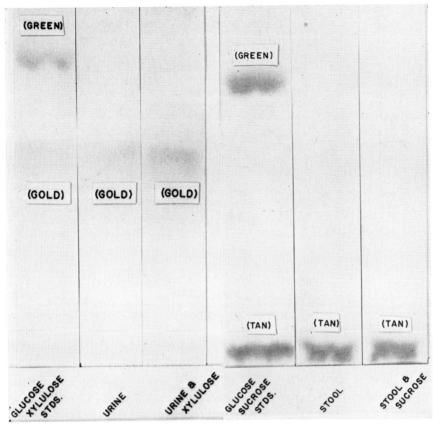

Fig. X-5.—High-voltage electrophoretograms showing individual sugars in (left) the urine of a patient with essential pentosuria, and (right) the stool of an infant convalescing from acute gastroenteritis.

QUANTITATION OF INDIVIDUAL SUGARS

The individual sugars are partitioned, developed, and identified as described in the preceding sections. Quantitation by means of comparisons with simultaneously run standards is desirable on occasion. To accomplish this, the standards and specimens must be applied as bands with a sample applicator.* They remain in bands during electrophoresis and development. The papers are cut into strips 3 cm. in width and scanned with a recording densitometer-integrator.† Appropriate interference filters are used for the different colors:

> 450 mμ for green bands
> 500 mμ for pink bands
> 570 mμ for purple or lavender bands
> 600 mμ for blue bands

---

*No. 300-805 Spinco Division of Beckman Instruments, Palo Alto, Calif.

†Model R.B. Analytrol manufactured by Spinco Division of Beckman Instruments, Inc., Palo Alto, Calif. Optical density cam (B-2) used.

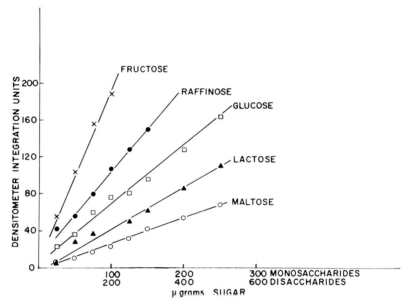

Fig. X-6.—Representative sugar proportionality data using diphenylamine-p-anisidine location reagent.

Scanning is facilitated by using neutral density filters to compensate for the backgrounds of the electrophoretic strips. The areas under the separate peaks are proportional to the color intensity and band widths; this is reflected in the integrator units recorded at the bottom of each tracing. Scanned strips are shown. Integration units are proportional to the concentration(s) of sugar(s) on the paper.

Quantities of individual sugars are calculated as follows:

$$\frac{\text{integration units of unknown}}{\text{integration units of standard}} \times \begin{array}{c}\text{quantity of standard}\\\text{on paper in m}\mu\\\text{moles or }\mu\text{g}\end{array} \times \begin{array}{c}\text{aliquot}\\\text{factor}\end{array} \times \begin{array}{c}\text{quantity of}\\\text{sugar/unit}\\\text{volume}\end{array}$$

REFERENCES

1. Ford, J. D., and Haworth, J. C.: The fecal excretion of sugars in children. J. Pediat. 63:988–990, 1963.

2. Gryboski, J. D., Zilis, J., and Ma, O. H.: A study of fecal sugars by high-voltage electrophoresis. Gastroenterloogy. 47:26–31, 1964.

3. Mabry, C. C., Gryboski, J. D., and Karam, E. A.: Rapid identification of mono- and oligosaccharides: An adaptation of high-voltage paper electrophoresis for sugars and its application to biologic materials. J. Lab. Clin. Med. 62:817–830, 1963.

CHAPTER XI

Mucopolysacchariduria

Clinical Annotation

COMPLEXES OF mucopolysaccharide-protein are normal constituents of connective tissue, cartilage, subcutaneous tissue, blood vessel walls, and the cornea. The metabolism of these substances is disturbed in disorders of connective tissues, the greatest alterations occurring in the so-called genetic mucopolysaccharidoses. They are characterized by abnormal and excessive tissue storage and urinary excretion of these substances. Only recently have these similar clinical states been delineated, each of which is a primary gene-determined disorder of mucopolysaccharide metabolism. The current classification is shown.

Collection Notes

For screening purposes, randomly voided urine is used. Mucopolysaccharide excretion varies throughout the day, so, for quantitative estimates, twenty-four hour collections of urine are used. Toluene with refrigeration (4° C.) is suitable for specimen preservation.

Interpretation of Results

Several laboratory tests have been devised to aid in diagnosis of the mucopolysaccharidoses, although none has received universal acceptance. We are using three screening tests that estimate total acid mucopolysaccharides in urine. Additional biochemical techniques for fractionation of the individual components of the acid mucopolysaccharides permits differentiation of the various genetic forms of the mucopolysaccharidoses. Normally, trace amounts of mucopolysaccharides are excreted in urine. Chondroitin sulfate A comprises about 80 per cent, with chondroitin sulfate B and heparatin sulfate accounting for the remainder. Mucopolysaccharide excretion may be greater in early life, thus care must be exercised in interpreting some screening tests. The semi-quantitative tests we use give definite three to four plus results with the urine of Type I patients, but less intense reactions with the other forms of the mucopolysaccaridoses. Slightly to moderately positive reactions with urine from unaffected patients may occur in association with urinary infections or unclean specimens. These positive reactions are due to an excess of mucoprotein.

METHODS

TOLUIDINE BLUE SPOT TEST

Principle

Certain cationic dyes shift their absorption spectrum toward shorter wavelengths in the presence of chemical substances with appropriately arranged

Table XI-1.—The Genetic Mucopolysaccaridoses

Proposed Designation	Pathologic Mucopolysacchariduria	Clinical Characteristics
Type I. (Hurler syndrome)	Chondroitin sulfate B (80%) and heparitin sulfate (20%)	Early clouding of cornea, liver and spleen greatly enlarged, severe bone deformities, stiff joints, mental retardation, prone to heart failure, usually die before puberty. 1:10,000; autosomal recessive.
Type II. (Hunter syndrome)	Chondroitin sulfate B (55%) and heparitin sulfate (45%)	Resembles Type I, but less severe. No clouding of cornea. Mental deterioration slow, and patients survive into middle life. $\approx$1:40,000; X-linked recessive.
Type III. (Sanfilippo syndrome)	Heparitin sulfate	Mental retardation dominates clinical features. No clinical clouding of cornea; incorstant fine corneal opacities. Hepatosplenomegaly and bone deformities mild. Very rare; autosomal recessive.
Type IV. (Morquio syndrome)	Keratosulfate	Severe and characteristic bone deformities dominate clinical features. Late clouding of cornea, hepatosplenomegaly slight, intellect probably normal, may have cardiac involvement. Survive into middle life. 1:40,000; autosomal recessive.
Type V. (Scheie syndrome)	Chondroitin sulfate B	Corneal clouding most dense peripherally, liver and spleen normal in size, bone deformities mild, stiff joints with carpal tunnel syndrome. Intellect probably normal. Develop aortic regurgitation. Survive into middle and late life. Very rare; autosomal recessive.
Type VI. (Maroteaux-Lamy syndrome)	Chondroitin sulfate B	Early clouding of cornea, hepatosplenomegaly, severe bone deformities, stiff joints, intellect normal, cardiac involvement. Very rare; autosomal recessive.

Other Types. There are other cases of the Hurler-like syndrome which defy categorization by the clinical, genetic, and biochemical methods now available. These usually have little or no increase in urinary mucopolysaccharide excretion.

Similar, But Non-mucopolysaccharide Conditions:

Familial neurovisceral lipidosis (Norman's disease)	Glycolipid	No clouding of cornea, hepatosplenomegaly, bone deformities moderate, mental retardation, death in infancy. Very rare; autosomal recessive.
Langer chondrodystrophy	Excess amount of acid mucoid material in urine (probably glycoprotein)	Corneal clouding by slit lamp exam, bone deformities moderately severe, intellect normal. Very rare; presumed autosomal recessive.

anionic groups. Correspondingly, light of a longer wavelength is transmitted. The phenomenon is termed metachromasia. Toluidine blue reacts with acid mucopolysaccharides to give this color change.

Reagents

1. *Sodium Acetate, 1M*

Sodium acetate	82.04 Gm.
Distilled water, q.s.	1000.00 ml.

   Dissolve the sodium acetate in distilled water and dilute to a volume of 1 L. Adjust to pH 2 with acetic acid.

2. *o-Toluidine Blue*

o-Toluidine blue	40 mg.
Sodium acetate, 1M, q.s.	100 ml.

   Dissolve the dye in 1M sodium acetate and dilute to volume.

3. *Standard*

Chondroitin sulfate	10 mg.
Distilled water, q.s.	100 ml.

   Dissolve the chondroitin sulfate in distilled water and dilute to a volume of 100 ml.

Procedure

1. Apply 50 and 100 μL. of urine on separate spots (no larger than 5 mm. in diameter) on a Whatman No. 1 filter paper. Use 5 μL. (0.5 μg) and 10 μL. (1 μg) of the dissolved chondroitin sulfate as visual standards.

2. Dip the paper for 1 minute in toluidine blue, drain, and rinse with 95 per cent ethyl alcohol.

Results

Urine with excess acid mucopolysaccharides gives a purple spot against a light blue background.

CETYLTRIMETHYLAMMONIUM BROMIDE TEST

Principle

Cetyltrimethylammonium bromide reacts with mucopolysaccharides to form an insoluble complex. This complex appears as a visible flocculent precipitate.

Reagents

1. *Citric Acid, 1M*

Citric acid	21.01 Gm.
Distilled water, q.s.	100.00 ml.

   Dissolve the sodium citrate in distilled water and dilute to volume.

2. *Sodium Citrate, 1M*

Sodium citrate ($C_6H_5O_7Na_8 \cdot 2H_2O$)	29.41 Gm.
Distilled water, q.s.	100.00 ml.

   Dissolve the sodium citrate in distilled water and dilute to volume.

3. *Citrate Buffer, pH6*

    Citric acid, 1M   9.5 ml.
    Sodium citrate, 1M   41.5 ml.
    Distilled water, q.s.   100.0 ml.

    Mix citric solutions and dilute to final volumes of 100 ml.

4. *Hexadecyltrimethylammonium Bromide*

    Hexadecyltrimethylammonium bromide   5 Gm.
    Citrate buffer pH 6   1000 ml.

    Dissolve bromide salt in citrate buffer and dilute to final volume.

Procedure

1. Pipet 5 ml. of clean, fresh urine at room temperature. Always use room temperature urine; a cold urine will give a positive test.
2. Add 1 ml. of hexadecyltrimethylammonium bromide.
3. Mix well by swirling and let stand at room temperature for 30 minutes.
4. Observe for heavy flocculent precipitate.

ACID ALBUMIN TURBIDITY TEST

Principle

A method previously developed for the assay of hyaluronidase has been modified for the detection of pathologic excesses of acid mucopolysaccharides excretion in dialyzed urine. It is based on the fact that these acidic polymers react with albumin at pH 3.75 to produce turbidity. Under appropriately controlled conditions of pH, ionic strength, temperature and time, this method can be used for approximate quantitation of the concentration of acid mucopolysaccharides.

Reagents

1. *Acid Albumin Reagent*

    Sodium acetate   16.3 Gm.
    Acetic acid, glacial   22.8 ml.
    Bovine albumin, fraction V   5.0 Gm.
    Distilled water, q.s.   5000.0 ml.

    Dissolve the sodium acetate in about 4 L. of distilled water. Add 22.8 ml. glacial acetic acid and mix well. Then dissolve the fraction V albumin in the solution and dilute to a volume of 5 L. Adjust pH to 3.75 with concentrated HCl (approximately 7 ml.). Filter through Whatman No. 1 filter paper and store in the refrigerator. Allow to come to room temperature prior to using in test procedure.

2. *Acid Albumin Blank Reagent*

    Sodium acetate   16.3 Gm.
    Acetic acid, glacial   22.8 ml.
    Distilled water, q.s.   5000.0 ml.

    Dissolve the sodium acetate in about 4 L. of distilled water. Add 22.8

glacial acetic acid and mix well. Dilute to final volume of 5 L. Adjust pH to 3.75 with concentrated HCl (approximately 8 ml.).

3. *Sodium Phosphate Buffer*

Sodium phosphate	42.6 Gm.
Sodium chloride	9.0 Gm.
Citric acid	30.0 Gm.
Distilled water, q.s.	1000.0 ml.

Dissolve dry ingredients in distilled water and dilute to final volume of 1 L.

4. *Standard Solution*

Chondroitin sulfate	50 mg.
Distilled water, q.s.	100 ml.

Dissolve the chondroitin sulfate in distilled water and dilute to final volume of 100 ml. Make dilutions in varying concentrations of 0.1 to 0.5 mg/ml. for use as working standards. The method of preparation of the mucopolysaccharides, their polymer size, and their qualitative character will affect the turbidity produced.

Apparatus

Apparatus needed for this procedure is dialysis tubing (Size 8 DC) and a standard clinical laboratory spectrophotometer.

Procedure

1. Pipet 6 ml. of well agitated urine (to mix the sediment uniformly) into a ¼ in. diameter Visking cellophane dialysis tube that has been tied in a knot at one end and checked for leakage with distilled water.

2. After tying off filled dialysis bag at the other end and labeling the specimen, dialyze for three to four hours in a volume of distilled water at least 150 times the volume of urine being dialyzed.

3. Upon completion of dialysis, transfer the contents of dialysis bag to a 15 ml. heavy walled centrifuge tube. Add enough distilled water to bring the volume of the sample to double its original volume, thus equalizing volume variations brought about by dialysis procedure.

4. After mixing, centrifuge for at least 10 minutes at maximum speed of clinical centrifuge to sediment any insoluble residues. Use only the clear supernatant for the turbidimetric measurement.

5. Set up reagents and specimens to be analyzed as follows in 25 by 105 mm. Coleman cuvets.

Tube No.	Sample	Sample Volume	Phosphate Buffer	Acid Albumin Reagent	Blank Acid Reagent
1	Distilled H$_2$O	1.5 ml.	0.5 ml.	10 ml.	—
2	Distilled H$_2$O	1.5 ml.	0.5 ml.	10 ml.	—
3	Unknown supernate	1.5 ml.	0.5 ml.	10 ml.	—
4	Unknown supernate	1.5 ml.	0.5 ml.	10 ml.	—
5	Unknown supernate	1.5 ml.	0.5 ml.	—	10 ml.
6	Unknown supernate	1.5 ml.	0.5 ml.	—	10 ml.

Unknown and phosphate buffer can be mixed prior to addition of the acid al-bumin reagent or the acid albumin reagent blank. Using a stop watch, add acid albumin reagent to each tube at 30 second intervals; shake tubes to assure proper mixing.

6. Exactly 10 minutes after addition of the acid albumin reagent, obtain the optical density reading at 600 mμ using a Coleman Jr. Spectrophotometer. The distilled water blank is used as the zero reference.

7. The average reading of Tubes 5 and 6 is subtracted from the average reading of Tubes 3 and 4. Use the resultant optical density reading as an estimate of the mucopolysaccharides present in the unknown sample.

Discussion

Tubes 5 and 6 with the acid albumin reagent blank are used to compensate for variation in urine pigment that could contribute to optical density. In several thousand tests on individuals with various types of growth and de-velopmental retardation, the only greatly elevated optical density measure-ments were obtained from individuals with the Hurler syndrome. Weakly positive reactions have been found in about one-third of newborn infants for the first forty-eight hours of life, and occasionally in hypothyroid children who had been started on thyroid treatment.

Sources of Error

The major source of error is contamination of the urine specimen with mucus from the genitourinary tract. This usually can be avoided or minimized if specimens less than 60 ml. in volume are *not* accepted for analysis.

Urine dilution factors can and do affect results; however, it must be em-phasized that this is only a rough quantitative screening procedure. This is a meaningful test only by virtue of the fact that individuals with the Hurler syndrome excrete so much more of these substances than do normal individuals.

Range of Values

Normal range is O.D. 0.00 to 0.02. Optical density values greater than 0.02 are usually indicative of excessive nondialyzable glycoprotein or mucopoly-saccharide polymers.

Clinical Interpretation of the Acetic Acid-Bovine Albumin Technique

Urine samples from individuals affected with the Hurler syndrome have O.D. values that range from 0.05 to 0.50. Only rarely have false negatives been obtained from these patients. Urine from children with hereditary mul-tiple exostoses or with the nail-patella syndrome may have O.D. values less than 0.03.

REFERENCES

1. Berry, H. K., and Spinanger, J.: A paper spot test useful in study of Hurler's syndrome. J. Lab. Clin. Med. 55:136–138, 1960.

2. Di Ferrante, N., and Rich, C.: Mucopolysaccharide of normal urine. Clin. Chem. Acta. 1:519–524, 1956.

3. Dorfman, A.: Studies on the biochemistry of connective tissue. Pediatrics. 22:576–589, 1958.

4. Dorfman, A., and Ott, M. L.: A turbidimetric method for the assay of hyaluronidase. J. Biol. Chem. 172:367–375, 1948.

5. Langer, Jr., L. O., Kronenberg, R. A., and Gorlin, R. J.: A case simulating Hurler syndrome of unusual longevity, without abnormal mucopolysacchariduria; A proposed classification of the various forms of the syndrome and similar diseases. Amer. J. Med. 40: 448–457, 1966.

6. Lorincz, A. E.: Measurements of urinary acid mucopolysaccharides. *In* Sunderman, F. W. (Ed.): Applied Seminar on the Clinical Pathology of Infancy. Philadelphia, Association of Clinical Pathology, 1965, pp. XVI, 1–4.

7. McKusick, V. A., Kaplan, D., Wise, D., Hanley, W. B., Suddarth, S. B., Sevick, M. E., and Maumanee, A. E.: The genetic mucopolysaccharidoses. Medicine. 44:445–483, 1965.

CHAPTER XII

Phenylketonuria Tests

Clinical Annotation

PHENYLKETONURIA is a Mendelian recessively inherited metabolic disorder which usually causes mental retardation and other neurologic deficits. However, our widening experience shows that some affected individuals may seem normal or only minimally affected. It occurs in about 1:10,000 births, and recent legislation requires testing of all infants at birth. A copy of the Kentucky law passed in 1966, and the resulting public health directives are shown. This law was prompted by the fact that early detection and adequate treatment will permit normal to near-normal mental development in the affected individual. The disorder is the result of deficient activity of phenylalanine hydroxylase, an enyzme found in the liver and necessary for the conversion of phenylalanine to tyrosine. When phenylalanine hydroxylase activity is deficient, oxidation of phenylalanine does not occur and phenylalanine accumulates in the blood. This results in an abnormal accumulation of otherwise normal metabolites; they appear in the urine after they become elevated in the plasma.

Collection Precautions

For these tests, plasma or serum as usually collected is suitable. For blood phenylalanine by mail, capillary blood may be submitted on Schleicher and Schuell No. 903 filter paper. Blood should saturate a 7/16 in. diameter circle; this requires 2 to 3 drops. The circle of blood is removed with a punch. The use of a punch insures uniform sampling.

Freshly voided urine, 5 to 10 ml., is submitted. It is important that the test be performed promptly or the urine stored frozen, because phenylpyruvic acid may deteriorate.

Interpretation of Results

Though there are many metabolic aberrations in phenylketonuria, the diagnosis can be established by the following laboratory criteria:

1. Blood, plasma, or serum phenylalanine concentration greater than 15 mg./100 ml.

2. Blood, plasma, or serum tyrosine concentration less than 5 mg./100 ml.

3. Urine phenylalanine concentration greater than 5 mg./100 ml.

4. Urine phenylpyruvic acid concentration greater than 15 mg./100 ml.

5. Urine o-hydroxyphenylacetic acid concentration greater than 0.25 mg./100 ml.

All of these findings do not regularly occur until the infant has received normal protein feedings (milk) for up to several weeks. This frequently is

COMMONWEALTH OF KENTUCKY

GENERAL ASSEMBLY

REGULAR SESSION, 1966

————————

HOUSE BILL NO. 164

————————

FRIDAY, FEBRUARY 11, 1966

————————

The following bill was reported to the Senate from the House and ordered to be printed.

AN ACT relating to testing infants for inborn errors of metabolism.

Be it enacted by the General Assembly of the Commonwealth of Kentucky:

(1) The administrative officer or other person in charge of each institution caring for infants twenty-eight days or less of age and the person required in pursuance of the provisions of KRS 213.050(1) shall register the birth of a child, and cause to have administered to every such infant or child in its or his care a test for inborn errors of metabolism in accordance with rules or regulations prescribed by the Commissioner of Health. Testing and the recording of the results of such tests shall be performed at such times and in such manner as may be prescribed by the Commissioner of Health.

(2) Nothing in this Act shall be construed to require the testing of any child whose parents are members of a nationally recognized and established church or religious denomination, the teachings of which are opposed to medical tests, and who object in writing to the testing of such child on that ground.

Fig. XII-1.—"PKU" law as passed in Kentucky.

the case for o-hydroxyphenylacetic acid. However, blood phenylalanine which is normally less than 2 mg./100 ml. will exceed 4 mg./100 ml. in an affected patient that has received either breast or bottle milk for forty-eight hours or more.

Factors which delay the appearance of derivative metabolites in an affected patient's urine include both the degree of hyperphenylalaninemia and

MCH - 3

TESTS FOR PHENYLKENTONURIA (PKU) OF NEWBORN BABIES

Relates to KRS 214.155

Pursuant to the authority of KRS 214.155

(1) Except as otherwise provided in subsection (2) of KRS 214.155, the administrative officer or other person in charge of each hospital or institution caring for infants 28 days or less of age and the attending physician or midwife shall cause to have administered to every newborn baby in its or his care a blood test to detect phenylkentonuria (PKU). In the event a baby is not born in a hospital or other institution, the attending physician or midwife shall be solely responsible for causing such test to be administered.

(2) Hospitals and institutions may submit blood samples to the Division of Laboratory Services, State Department of Health, where tests shall be performed without charge or they may elect to conduct their own testing program, in which event the State Department of Health shall be so notified and the laboratory procedure shall be approved. The laboratory may be required by the State Department of Health to demonstrate its proficiency in the performance of the test. Positive results of tests shall be reported within 24 hours to the Director of Mental Retardation, State Department of Health, and to the physician concerned.

Adopted: May 26, 1966
Filed: June 22, 1966
Effective: July 22, 1966

Figs. XII-2 (above), XII-3, and XII-4.—Public Health Department directives for implementing "PKU" law.

the maturity of the individual phenylalanine degradation enzymes in the liver. In the untreated older patient, all of these metabolites may be found in ten- to fiftyfold excess. In the affected patient under dietary care, an attempt is made to keep the phenylalanine level less than 8 mg. per cent. The ferric chloride test for phenylpyruvic acid in urine does not become positive until the phenylalanine concentration in the blood attains a value of 12 mg. per cent or more.

COMMONWEALTH OF KENTUCKY
DEPARTMENT OF HEALTH
275 EAST MAIN STREET
FRANKFORT, KENTUCKY – 40601

M E M O R A N D U M

August 1, 1966

TO: All Practicing Physicians and Hospital Administrators
          All County Health Departments

FROM: Russell E. Teague, M. D., MPH

SUBJECT: Phenylketonuria (PKU) Testing Law and Regulation

A new state law (HB No. 164) is now effective which makes PKU testing of newborn infants compulsory.

As you will recall, we have had a statewide "voluntary" blood testing screening program for PKU since December 1965 in which more than half of our Kentucky hospitals have participated.

Now that the new PKU law, which was introduced by a lay group, has become effective, we intend to make a concerted effort, with your assistance, to make the program a success.

I am enclosing a copy of HB No. 164 and the regulation promulgated thereunder. I believe that the regulation fully sets forth the responsibilities, requirements and procedures involved.

Please note that the urine test is not acceptable and that only the blood test is presently approved. However, the blood test is not accurate until 24 to 48 hours after the infant has been started on milk feeding. Therefore, the test should not be obtained prior to 48 to 72 hours of life.

Please feel free to inquire if you have questions regarding the program.

Russell E. Teague, M. D., MPH
Commissioner of Health

Attachment

Fig. XII-3.

PHENYLALANINE (Blood, Plasma, Serum)

Principle

The method depends on the fluorescence of a phenylalanine-ninhydrin reaction product. Its sensitivity is due to the presence of the dipeptide, glycyl-1-leucine, which enhances the reaction between phenylalanine and ninhydrin. The reaction takes place at pH of 5.8, a pH at which other amino acids will not react with ninhydrin. Fluorescence is excited with 350 mμ to 365 mμ light; the

MCH 3

TESTS FOR PHENYLKETONURIA (PKU) OF NEWBORN BABIES

Relates to KRS 214.155

Pursuant to the authority of KRS 214.155

(1) Except as otherwise provided in subsection (2) of KRS 214.155,
the administrative officer or other person in charge of each hospital
or institution caring for infants 28 days or less of age and the
attending physician or midwife shall cause to have administered to
every newborn baby in its or his care a blood test to detect phenylketonuria
(PKU). In the event a baby is not born in a hospital or other institution,
the attending physician or midwife shall be solely responsible for causing
such test to be administered.

(2) Hospitals and institutions may submit blood samples to the
Division of Laboratory Services, State Department of Health, where tests
shall be performed without charge or they may elect to conduct their
own testing program, in which event the State Department of Health shall
be so notified and the laboratory procedure shall be approved. The
laboratory may be required by the State Department of Health to demonstrate its proficiency in the performance of the test. Positive results
of tests shall be reported within 24 hours to the Director of Mental
Retardation, State Department of Health, and to the physician concerned.

****

The undersigned, Russell E. Teague, states that he is Secretary
of the State Board of Health and that the foregoing regulation was
duly adopted by the State Board of Health at a meeting held at Frankfort,
Kentucky, on the _____day of_____, 1966.

Witness my hand and seal of office this the _____day of
_____, 1966.

_____
Russell E. Teague, M.D.
Secretary
Kentucky State Board of Health

****

Fig. XII-4.

emitted visible light has maximum absorption in a broad area, 485 mμ to 530
mμ, of the light spectrum.

MICROAUTOMATED METHOD

Preparation of Reagents

1. *Saline*

Sodium chloride	9 Gm.
Chloroform	2 Gm.
Distilled water, q.s.	1000 ml.

HOSPITAL PKU BLOOD TEST

Fill in all information with *pencil* only:

HOSPITAL

Baby's Name
_____

_____

Date of birth ....

Date 1st feeding ....

Bottle ☐;   Breast ☐;   Both ☐

Date of Sample ....

Premature?   Yes ☐;   No ☐
Baby's Doctor

....

Doctor's Address:

Kentucky State Department of Health
PKU SCREENING PROGRAM

INSTRUCTIONS FOR COLLECTING
BLOOD SAMPLE

After the skin is sterilized, the infant's heel is punctured with a sterile disposable lancet. If bleeding is slow, it is helpful to hold the limb dependent for a short period before spotting the blood on the filter paper. To insure an adequate test, each circle on the filter paper must be *filled completely* with a large drop of blood which has *soaked through* the paper. This can best be done by placing *this* side of the filter paper against the baby's heel and watching for the blood to appear on the front side of the paper and completely fill the circle.

The blank spaces are filled in with pencil (ball point pen or regular ink blurs and becomes illegible in the autoclaving that precedes the testing).

Only positive or suspicious results will be reported.

FILL 3 CIRCLES WITH BLOOD
(Be sure blood soaks through.)

Fig. XII-5.—Front and back of filter paper used for collection of capillary blood for phenylalanine measurements.

Add sodium chloride to a volumetric flask containing 600 ml. of distilled water. Add 2 ml. of chloroform. Dilute to volume and mix. Add 0.5 ml. of Brij.-35.

2. *Stock Succinate Buffer: 1 M pH 5.8 ± 0.1*

Succinic acid	118.0 Gm.
Sodium hydroxide	68.6 Gm.
Distilled water, q.s.	1000.0 ml.

Slowly add the succinic acid to about 500 ml. of distilled water, stirring constantly with a magnetic mixer in a 1 L. volumetric flask. When the acid is in solution, slowly add the sodium hydroxide. Allow to cool to room temperature and dilute to volume. Check the pH carefully, using 6N sodium hydroxide or 6N hydrochloric acid to bring to pH 5.8 ± 0.1. Keep refrigerated when not in use.

3. *Working Succinate Buffer: 0.04M pH 5.8 ± 0.1*

Stock succinate buffer	40 ml.
Distilled water, q.s.	1000 ml.

Add stock buffer to a 1 L. volumetric flask. Dilute to volume with distilled water and mix well. Adjust pH using 0.1 N HCl or 0.1 N NaOH to pH 5.8±0.1. Add 1 ml. of Brij.-35 and mix. Keep refrigerated when not in use.

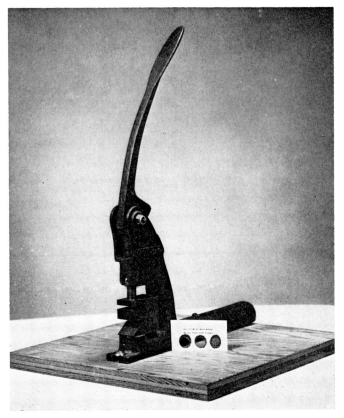

Fig. XII-6.—Mechanical punch for obtaining uniform 7/16 in. diameter filter paper circles impregnated with blood.

Table XII-1.—Percentage of 104 PKU Urine Samples Giving Definitely
Positive Reactions after Intervals of Exposure at Room Temperature

Exposure Time (Hours)	FeCl$_3$ (Test Tube)	Dinitrophenylhydrazine (DNPH)	Phenistix (Filter Paper)
2	99.1	100	99.1
4	95.2	100	98.1
8	95.2	100	98.1
12	95.3	100	97.1
18	90.4	100	96.2
24	76.0	100	91.3

From a report to the Technical Committee on Clinic Programs for Mentally Retarded Children, Washington, D.C., February 26-27, 1959.

4. Ninhydrin

Ninhydrin   5.34 Gm.
Distilled water, q.s.   1000.00 ml.

Place ninhydrin in a 1 L. volumetric flask containing 800 ml. of distilled water. Stir with magnetic mixer until all ninhydrin is in solution.

This may take several hours. Dilute to volume, mix and store in an amber bottle in refrigerator.

NOTE: Solution will stain skin purple. Avoid contact.

5. *Glycyl-1-leucine*

Glycyl-1-leucine	100 mg.
Distilled water, q.s.	100 ml.

Place 100 mg. of glycyl-1-leucine in 100 ml. volumetric flask. Dilute to volume with 100 ml. distilled water and mix well. Store in a refrigerator.

6. *Copper Reagent*

Sodium carbonate	16.00 Gm.
Potassium sodium tartarate	0.65 Gm.
Cupric sulfate with 5 H_2O	0.60 Gm.
Distilled water, q.s.	1000.00 ml.

Dissolve the sodium carbonate in 300 ml. of distilled water. Dissolve the tartarate in 300 ml. of distilled water. Dissolve the copper sulfate in 300 ml. of water. Add the tartarate solution to carbonate solution in a 1 L. volumetric flask. Add the cupric solution, dilute to volume with water, and mix well.

7. *Stock Standard*

L-phenylalanine	50.00 mg.
NaCl	0.45 Gm.
Distilled water, q.s.	50.00 ml.

Dissolve 50 mg. of carefully weighed 1-phenylalanine in about 10 ml. of warm isotonic saline in a 50 ml. volumetric flask. Dilute to volume.

8. *Working Standards: Aqueous, In-serum or In-blood*

Expected Value (mg.%)	Stock Phenylalanine (ml.)	qs to Volume with Either Water, Serum or Blood
2	1.0	qs 50 ml.
4	2.0	qs 50 ml.
6	3.0	qs 50 ml.
8	4.0	qs 50 ml.
12	6.0	qs 50 ml.
16	8.0	qs 50 ml.
20	10.0	qs 50 ml.

"In-serum" standards are separated into 0.5 ml. aliquots and stored frozen. Also, there is an additional 1 to 2 mg. per cent naturally occurring in the sera used to prepare the standards.

For blood phenylalanine measurements from filter paper, submitted by mail, "in-blood" standards are prepared using outdated blood-bank blood as above. Care should be taken to moisten only a 7/16 in. diameter circle of the filter paper; larger amounts oversaturate the paper and cause spuriously high standard measurements. These on-paper standards may be stored at room temperature for up to six months.

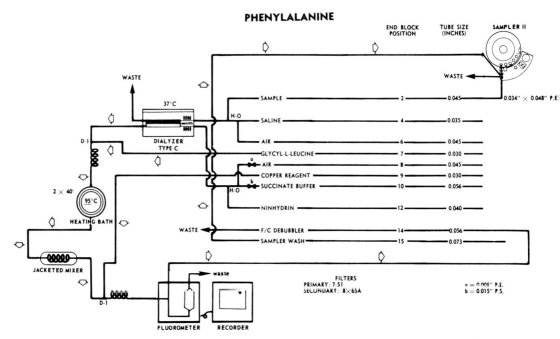

Fig. XII-7.—Flow diagram for phenylalanine (blood, plasma, or serum).

Apparatus

A basic AutoAnalyzer unit using a double 40-foot heating bath is employed with a fluorometer in place of a colorimeter.

Operating Notes

1. Turn recorder module to "on" position by moving top toggle switch on unit. Let warm up for at least 15 minutes.

2. Turn the fluorometer on by toggle switch on unit. Let warm up for at least 15 minutes.

3. Stretch manifold blocks to first or second notches and lock pump rollers on platen. Pump distilled water for about 20 minutes.

4. Push light for fluorescent light to be activated; allow to warm up.

5. Adjust recorder base line at 10 per cent transmission by means of the "blank" dial on the fluorometer.

6. Place reagent lines in respective working reagent bottles and pump for about 20 minutes.

7. Using 60/hr. sampler cam, sample a high standard eluted from filter paper or a 1 mg. per cent aqueous phenylalanine standard; set recorder peak height between 70 and 80 per cent transmission. Place standards and samples on the platter. Situate platter on sampler with first standard or sample opposite sampling probe. Keep platter covered during sampling.

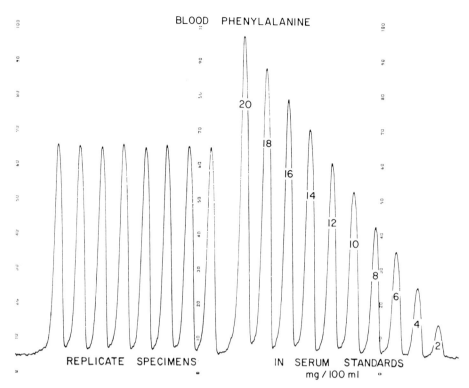

Fig. XII-8.—Phenylalanine recorder tracing; sample volume 0.1 ml. for both "in-serum" standards and patient specimens.

8. Serum, plasma, or whole blood specimen preparation: Run specimens at the rate of 60/hr. On the serum, plasma, or whole blood specimen, a dilution of 1:10 is made in the sample cup.

9. When blood phenylalanine measurements on finger-tip blood collected on filter paper are made, standards and specimens are obtained by making a 7/16 in. punch of special Schleicher and Schuell Co. filter paper which has previously been saturated with either in-blood standard or finger-tip blood specimen. The volume of in-blood standard and specimens are approximately 20 μL., but this need not be considered in comparison of standards and specimens (test) results. For reproducible and equivalent elution of phenylalanine from the filter paper punches, each punch must be handled the same. We have found the following to be convenient: Place each paper punch in separate 2 ml. centrifuge tubes. Add 1 ml. distilled water. Mix each tube mechanically on an agitator for 15 seconds. Let stand for 5 minutes. Repeat mechanical agitation for 30 seconds, decant eluate into sample cup. *Do not allow elution to occur for more than 10 minutes*, for irregularities occur with passive elution.

10. On the sample platter, standards and specimens are alternated with water cups. This permits an excellent wash between each specimen. An alternate method is to remove alternate "ears" on 60/hr. sampler cam.

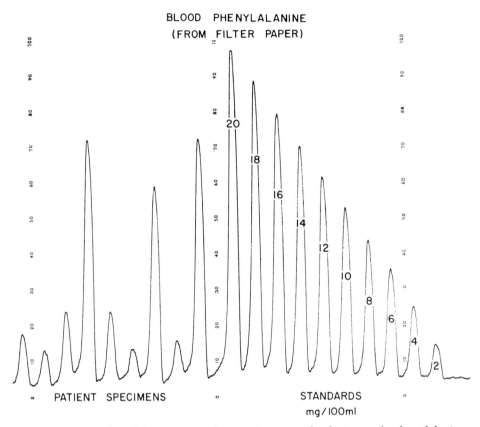

Fig. XII-9.—Phenylalanine recorder tracing; rapid elutions of phenylalanine from filter paper obtained for both "in-blood" standards and patient specimens.

Calculations

Sample chart recorder tracing of capillary blood specimens submitted by mail is shown. A curve is prepared from the apices of the standard peaks, and sample peaks are compared on this curve.

MICROMANUAL METHOD

Preparation of Reagents

1. *Trichloroacetic Acid: 0.6N*

Trichloroacetic acid	98 Gm.
Distilled water, q.s.	1000 ml.

   Dissolve the trichloroacetic acid in distilled water and dilute to 1 L. To obtain 0.3 N trichloroacetic acid for the blank and for making standards, 0.6 N trichloroacetic acid is diluted with an equal volume of water.

2. *Succinate Buffer: pH 5.8*

Sodium succinate • 2 H_2O	5.94 Gm.
Hydrochloric acid, 1N	4.00 ml.
Distilled water, q.s.	100.00 ml.

Table XII-2.—Fluorometers and Filter Combinations for Fluorometric
Measurement of Phenylalanine

Instrument	Primary	Secondary
Ferrand model A	Corning glass filter No. 5860 (365mµ)	No. 4304 and 3384 (505 to 530 mµ)
Turner model 110	Corning No. 7-51 (365 mµ) or Corning No. 7-60 (350 mµ)	Wratten No. 8 plus Wratten No. 65A (510 mµ)
Coleman Fluorometer model 12C	Narrow-pass filter with peak	Sharp-cut filter starting transmission at 485 mµ

Dissolve the sodium succinate in distilled water. Add the 1N hydrochloric acid, then dilute to 100 ml. with water. Adjust the pH to 5.8 (±0.1) with 1N HCl or 1N NaOH. The buffer should be stored in the refrigerator.

3. *Ninhydrin: (30mM)*

Ninhydrin	0.534 Gm.
Distilled water, q.s.	100.000 ml.

Dissolve ninhydrin in water and dilute to the volume of 100 ml. The reagent is stored in a brown bottle at room temperature.

4. *Glycyl-1-leucine: 5 mM*

Glycyl-1-leucine	0.941 Gm.
Distilled water, q.s.	100.000 ml.

Dissolve the glycyl-1-leucine in water and dilute to 100 ml. This reagent should be dispensed into small vials or tubes in approximately 1 ml. aliquots and stored in the deep freeze.

5. *Copper Reagent*

Sodium carbonate	1.60 Gm.
Potassium sodium tartarate	0.10 Gm.
Copper sulfate	0.06 Gm.
Distilled water, q.s.	1000.00 ml.

Dissolve separately in about 300 ml. of water each the sodium carbonate, potassium sodium tartarate, and copper sulfate. Mix the sodium carbonate and tartarate solutions together, then add the copper sulfate, and make up the volume to 1 L. This prevents precipitation of the cupric ions in alkaline solution. Keep reagent at room temperature.

6. *Standard Solutions*

In-serum standard solutions are prepared as described for the micro-automated method.

Apparatus

A suitable fluorometer with proper cuvets and filters, a water bath at 60° C., and a microcentrifuge are required. Satisfactory instruments and filter combinations are as shown.

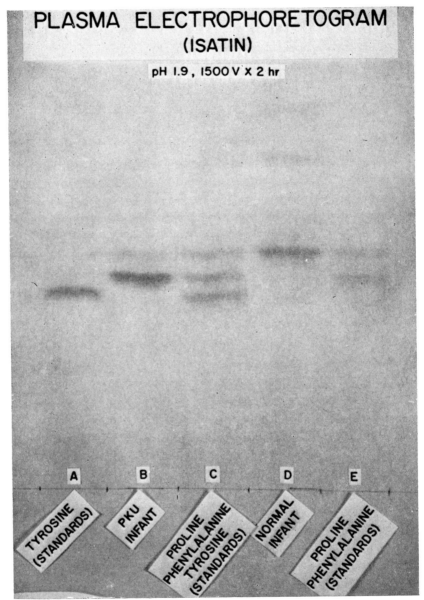

Fig. XII-10.—High-voltage paper electrophoretogram of plasma using location reagent (isatin) relatively selective for tyrosine, phenylalanine, and proline. Note great excess of phenylalanine and no detectable tyrosine in specimen from 10 day old PKU infant.

Procedure Notes:

1. Deproteinize serum or heparinized plasma by mixing equal quantities (0.05 ml. or more) of sample and 0.6 N trichloroacetic acid. Allow the mixture to stand for approximately 10 minutes, then centrifuge (about 2000 rpm) for 10 minutes.

2. While samples are centrifuging, prepare mixed reagent by adding together succinate buffer, ninhydrin, and leucylalanine in the volume of 10:4:2. (0.8 ml. of the mixture is required for each sample, blank or standard.)

3. In small tubes, mix 0.80 ml. of mixed reagent with 0.05 ml. supernatant (from deproteinization of sample), or standard working solution, or 0.3 N trichloroacetic acid (for the blank).

4. After thorough mixing, incubate the tubes in a water bath at 60° C. for two hours.

5. Cool tubes in an ice bath and add 5 ml. of copper reagent to each. Mix tube contents thoroughly and allow to stand at room temperature for 10 to 15 minutes.

6. Measure the fluorescence of the standards and samples after setting the blank at zero fluorescence. Primary (activating) wavelength is 365 $m\mu$ and the secondary (fluorescing) wavelength is 510 $m\mu$ (or filters closest to these wavelengths).

7. Potential sources of error of this method include (a) obtaining blood too early in life, (b) sampling postprandial bloods that show some elevation of serum phenylalanine, (c) inaccurate measurements of sample or reagents, (d) disregarding directions (prolonged heating or cooling time), (e) use of unstable reagents. (Leucylalanine must be discarded at the end of the day's run and should not be refrozen.)

Results and Calculations

Phenylalanine concentration is calculated from a standard curve, plotting fluorescence against phenylalanine concentration of the standards.

TYROSINE AND PHENYLALANINE, BLOOD AND URINE:
Measurement by High Voltage Paper Electrophoresis (HVPE)

The concentrations of phenylalanine and tyrosine may be measured simultaneously in biologic fluids by HVPE and subsequent development with isatin. The fluorescent method for phenylalanine in blood is not suitable for urine since urine usually contains substances that spuriously quench or enhance fluorescence.

The HVPE technique for identification and measurement of phenylalanine and tyrosine in biologic fluids is described in Chapter IX. Sample electrophoretograms of plasma and urine are shown.

URINE PHENYLPYRUVIC ACID

Principle

Qualitative tests for the presence of excess phenylpyruvic acid include the ferric chloride and the 2,4-dinitrophenylhydrazine (2,4-DNPH) reactions. Precise identification of phenylpyruvic acid is made by high-voltage electrophore-

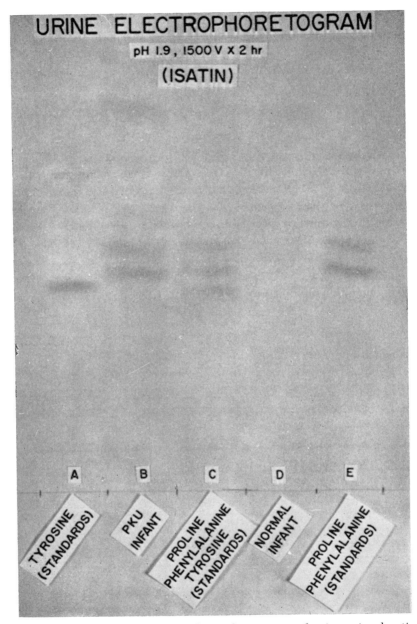

Fig. XII-11.—High-voltage paper electrophoretogram of urine using location re-agent relatively selective for tyrosine, phenylalanine, and proline. Note great excess of pheynlalanine and no detectable tyrosine in specimen from 10 day old PKU infant.

sis of urine and subsequent development of phenylpyruvic acid as a 2,4-dinitro-phenylhydrazone. Ferric chloride reacts to give a colored complex based on ferric ions combining wtih phenols and aliphatic enols. 2,4 DNPH reacts with ketoacids to form yellow precipitates.

Preparation of Reagents

    1. *Ferric Chloride*

Ferric chloride	10 Gm.
Distilled water, q.s.	100 ml.

        Dissolve ferric chloride in distilled water and dilute to 100 ml. volume. Solution must be stored in plastic bottle.

    2. *Dinitrophenylhydrazine*

2,4-dinitrophenylhydrazine (DNPH)	100 mg.
Hydrochloric acid, conc.	15 ml.
Distilled water	85 ml.

        Add water to DNPH and mix. Add concentrated hydrochloric acid. Shake in a shaking machine for 30 min. Allow to settle and use supernatant.

    3. *Sodium Carbonate*

Sodium carbonate	10 Gm.
Distilled water, q.s.	100 ml.

        Dissolve Na_2CO_3 in distilled water and dilute to 100 ml.

Procedure Notes

$FeCl_3$ Test. To 1 to 5 ml. of urine add 3 to 10 drops of 10 per cent ferric chloride. NOTE: It is not necessary to acidify the urine since the acidity of the $FeCl_3$ solution (pH: 1.8) counteracts any excess alkalinity of the urine. Observe for an immediate green color reaction; in a weakly positive reaction the color may fade in less than a half minute. Phenistix* may be used as an alternative technique, but positive reactions should be rechecked with the aqueous ferric chloride test.

2,4-DNPH Test. To 1 ml. of urine add 4 ml. of 0.1 per cent 2,4-dinitrophenylhydrazine. In a positive test a yellow precipitate is formed. Should a yellow precipitate form, more exact identification can be accomplished as follows: Wait 10 minutes; extract the precipitate with ether; then extract the ether with 10 per cent sodium carbonate. The yellow 2,4-dinitrophenylhydrazones of the ketoacids enter the water phase and develop a deep red color after the addition of an equal volume of 1 N sodium hydroxide.

For identification of phenylpyruvic acid by high-voltage paper electrophoresis, apply urine directly to the filter paper as for amino acids (Chapter IX). Partition the ketoacids at 2000 v for one hour along with suitable standards. Dry the paper in a vented chromatography oven at 90° C. for 30 minutes; then dip paper through a saturated solution of 2,4-dinitrophenylhydrazine in ethanol. Allow to dry at room temperature for 5 minutes, then redip paper through a 5 per cent solution of potassium hydroxide in ethanol. The ketoacids can be identified by their positions and characteristic color reactions.

---

*Phenistix is the registered trademark of the Ames Laboratory. The ferric chloride is buffered with cyclohexysulfamic acid; and magnesium ions have been added to minimize interference by phosphates.

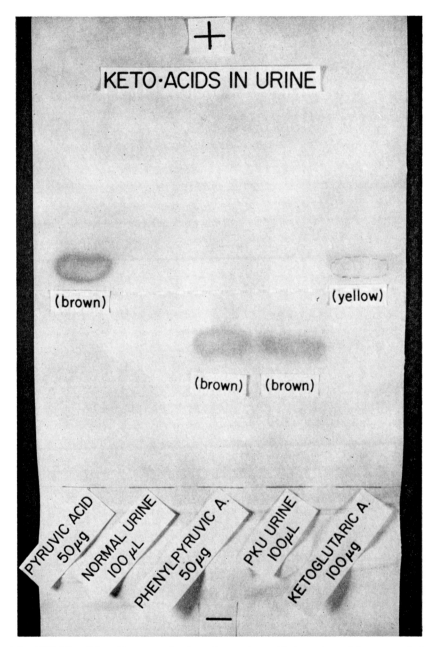

Fig. XII-12.—Identification of phenylpyruvic acid in urine. The normal keto-acids that occur in trace amounts are pyruvic, ketoglutaric and acetoacetic acids. Electrophoresis performed using pyridine-acetic buffer (pH 5.3) at a potential of 1500 v for 45 minutes. Locating of bands accomplished by sequential dipping in ethanolic solutions of 2,4-DNPH (saturated) and KOH (5 per cent).

Table XII-3.—Reactants in Ferric Chloride Tests

Substance	Color Produced with	
	Ferric Chloride Solution	Phenistix
Phenylpyruvic acid	Green or blue-green eventually fading	Gray-green or blue green, max. 1 min., fade slowly
p-hydroxyphenyl pyruvic acid	Green, fades in seconds	Green, fades in seconds
o-hydroxyphenyl pyruvic acid	Initial red-brown turning green or blue	Green, max. at 1 min.
o-hydroxyphenyl acetic acid	Mauve	Very pale mauve
Acetoacetic acid	Red or red-brown	Nil
Pyruvic acid	Deep gold yellow	Gold yellow
Homogentisic acid	Blue or green, fades quickly	Nil, brown with more concentrated solution
3-hydroxyanthranilic acid	Immediate deep brown	Yellow, turns green at 1 min., later brown
Salicylates	Stable purple	Stable purple
p-aminosalicylic acid	Red-brown	Pink to purple
Phenol derivs.	Violet	Nil
Vanillic acid	Red-mauve, turns deep brown	Brown
Xanthurenic acid	Deep green, later brown	Nil
α-ketobutyric acid	Purple, fades to red-brown	Faint brown-purple
Maple syrup disease urine	Gray with green tinge	Nil
Phenothiazine derivs. (Compazine, Thorazine)	Purple	?
Bilirubin	Blue-green	?
Antipyrines and acetophenetidines	Red	?
Imidazolepyruvic acid	Green or blue-green	Gray-green or blue-green

Results and Calculations

The green ferric chloride reaction is not unique for phenylpyruvic acid. It also gives variable colors with other substances. Interfering precipitates that occur are various salts, usually phosphates. For the 2,4-dinitrophenylhydrazine of phenylpyruvic acid, the precipitate formed is a canary yellow for both tests, and the intensity of the colors formed are proportionate to the concentration of phenylpyruvic acid. Both the ferric chloride and 2,4-dinitrophenylhydrazine reactions become positive (1+) when phenylpyruvic acid is present in a concentration of about 15 mg./100 ml. A strongly positive reaction (4+) corresponds to a concentration of about 100 mg./100 ml.

ORTHO-HYDROXYPHENYLACETIC ACID (o-HPAA)

Principles

Urine and o-HPAA standards are applied to filter paper at separate locations. The specimens are partitioned by descending paper chromatography. When the supporting filter paper is dried, the o-HPAA spots are developed with a specific locating reagent. The intensity of the individual spots are proportional to their concentrations. Visual comparisons between o-HPAA standards and o-HPAA in urine are made.

Preparation of Reagents

1. *Solvent for Chromatographic Partitioning*

		ml.	ml.	ml.
Isopropyl alcohol	20 parts	200	400	600
Ammonia	1 part	10	20	30
Distilled water	2 parts	20	40	60

2. *Standards*

Dissolve 10 mg. o-HPAA in 50 ml. water for a concentration of 200 μg/ml. Store 2 ml. labeled aliquots in freezer for future use.

$$\text{Molar conversion} \quad \frac{\text{gravimetric wt./vol.}}{\text{mol. wt.}} = \frac{10/50\ \text{ml.}}{152.1} = \frac{.2\ \text{mg./ml.}}{152.1}$$

$$= \frac{200\ \mu\text{g/ml.}}{152.1} = 1.314\ \mu\ \text{moles/ml.}$$

3. *Developing Reagent*

Dilute ethanolic solution of 2,6-dibromoquinone chlorimide followed by exposure to ammonia vapors.

a. 2,6-dibromoquinone chlorimide   0.1 Gm.
   Ethanol, 100 per cent   100.0 ml.
b. Ammonia (NH_4OH), conc.

Apparatus

The only special equipment required is a chromatography tank fitted for descending chromatography.

Procedure Notes

1. Preparation of paper: Use $22\frac{1}{2}'' \times 78\frac{1}{4}''$ Whatman No. 1 paper. Arrange specimens and standards as spots on origin lines as shown below. Accurately pipet specimens on to Whatman's No. 1 filter paper on origin line about $1\frac{1}{2}$ in. apart. Make spots no larger than 0.25 in. in diameter. Along with standards, use both negative and positive controls with each run. Suggested volumes of standards are 5.10 and 20 μL.; suggested volumes of urine specimens are 25 to 100 μL.

2. Partitioning of compounds: Place papers in tank with origin near the solvent trough. Allow solvent partitioning to occur by descending chromatography for six hours. Dry papers in oven at 60° C. for 15 minutes.

3. Color development of compounds: Dip dried paper through dilute 2,6-dibromoquinone chlorimide solution and allow to dry at room temperature. Expose to ammonia fumes in ventilated hood. Estimate intensity of blue spots and compare with standards.

Results and Calculations

o-hydroxyphenylacetic acid excretion is calculated as follows:

1. μg o-HPAA/ml. or mg. o-HPAA/100 ml.

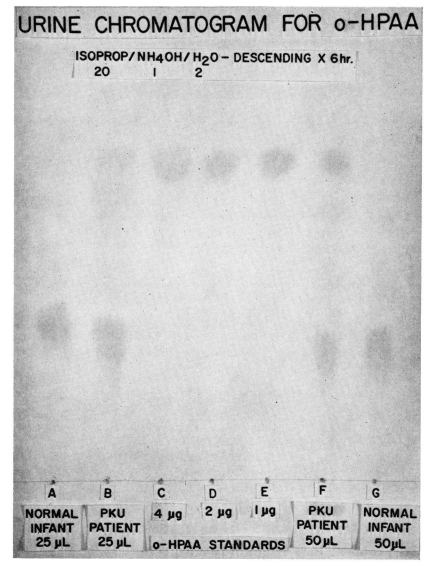

Fig. XII-13.—Rapid paper chromatographic separation and identification of ortho-hydroxyphenylacetic acid. Note large excess of o-HPAA in specimen from 10 day old PKU infant.

2.

$$\text{Equivalent amount } (\mu g) \text{ of o-HPAA in specimen} \times \frac{100}{\text{volume of specimen applied}} \times \frac{1}{152.1} = \mu \text{ moles o-HPAA/} 100 \text{ ml. urine}$$

3. Express o-HPAA as μ moles/Gm. creatinine

Obtain creatinine measurement on each urine, and twenty-four hour volume when possible. Usually, creatinine measurement is in mg./100 ml. Be sure to convert to Gm./100 ml.

$$\frac{\text{Gm. creatinine}}{100 \text{ ml.}} \times \frac{\mu \text{ moles o-HPAA}}{100 \text{ ml.}} = \mu \text{ moles/Gm. creatinine}$$

REFERENCES

1. Ambrose, J. A., Ingerson, A., Garrettson, L. G., and Chung, C. W.: A study of the fluoremetric method for phenylalanine in serum samples. Clin. Chim. Acta. 15:493–503, 1967.

2. Armstrong, M. D., Shaw, K. N. F., and Robinson, K. S.: Studies on phenylketonuria: II. Excretion of o-hydroxyphenylacetic acid in phenylketonuria. J. Biol. Chem. 213:797–804, 1955.

3. Berry, H. K., Sutherland, B. S., and Umbarger, B.: Detection of phenylketonuria in newborn infants. J.A.M.A. 198:1114–1115, 1966.

4. Berry, H. K., Sutherland, B. S., and Umbarger, B.: Diagnosis and treatment: Interpretation of results of blood screening studies for detection of phenylketonuria. Pediatrics. 37:102–106, 1966.

5. Centerwall, W. R., Berry, H. K., and Woolf, L. I.: In Lynan, F. L. (Ed.): Testing Methods in Phenylketonuria. Springfield, Charles C Thomas, 1963, pp. 123–130.

6. Clark, P. T., and Rice, J. D.: The use of filter paper PKU test specimen cards in the automated determination of blood phenylalanine concentration. Amer. J. Clin. Path. 46: 486–489, 1966.

7. Free, A. H., and Free, H. M.: Fluorimetric measurement of phenylalanine in serum. In Sunderman, F. W. (Ed.): Applied Seminar on the Clinical Pathology of Infancy. Philadelphia, Association of Clinical Pathology, 1965, pp. IV, 1–5.

8. Guthrie, R., and Susi, A.: A simple phenylalanine method for detecting phenylketonuria in large populations of newborn infants. Pediatrics. 32:338–343, 1963.

9. Hill, J. B., Summer, G. K., and Hill, H. D.: Modifications of the automated procedure for blood phenylalanine. Clin. Chem. 13:77–80, 1967.

10. Hill, J. B., Summer, G. K., Pender, M. W., and Roszel, N. O.: An automated procedure for blood phenylalanine. Clin. Chem. 11:541–546, 1965.

11. Hill, J. B., Summer, G. K., Shavender, E. F., Scurletis, R. D., Robie, W. A., Maddry, L. G., Matherson, M. S., and Brooks, M. F.: Early experience in use of automation in screening of phenylketonuria in a newborn population. In Skeggs Jr., L. T. (Ed.): Automation in Analytical Chemistry, Technicon Symposia, 1965. New York, Mediad, Inc., 1966, pp. 404–405.

12. Mabry, C. C., and Todd, W. R.: Quantitative measurement of individual and total free amino acids in urine; rapid method employing high-voltage paper electrophoresis and direct densitometry and its application to the urinary excretions of amino acids in normal subjects. J. Lab. Clin. Med. 61:146–157, 1963.

13. Mabry, C. C., and Karam, E. A.: Measurement of free amino acids in plasma and serum by high-voltage paper electrophoresis. Amer. J. Clin. Path. 42:421–430, 1964.

14. Kleinman, D. S., Twiss, S., and Day, R. W.: Some factors affecting McCaman-Robins test results in screening newborns for PKU. Pediatrics. 38:619–628, 1966.

15. McCaman, M. W., and Robins, E.: Fluorimetric method for the determination of phenylalanine in serum. J. Lab. Clin. Med. 59:885–890, 1962.

16. Tashian, R. E.: Phenylpyruvic acid as a possible precursor of o-hydroxyphenylacetic acid in man. Science. 129:1553, 1959.

CHAPTER XIII

Sweat Chloride

Clinical Annotation

OVER A DECADE AGO it was demonstrated that the sweat concentrations of sodium and chloride are greatly elevated in patients with cystic fibrosis of the pancreas. Shortly thereafter a practical test was introduced wherein the patient was placed in a plastic bag. The elicitation of sweat by this or other thermal means may be dangerous. There have been seven recorded deaths of infants who have been partially enclosed in plastic for thermal sweating. For these, as well as technical reasons, the iontophoretic method which chemically stimulates the formation of eccrine sweat is the preferred method.

Collection Precautions

Failure to obtain adequate amounts of sweat, 100 mg. or more, occurs not infrequently. These instances usually occur with premature or very young infants and with dehydrated or malnourished infants. Warming the baby and forcing fluids for several hours, then repeating the test may produce adequate amounts of sweat. Electrical burns may occur if the polarity of the current is reversed, if the current is increased above 5 ma., or if poorly conducting electrodes are used. Errors may arise from evaporation of water from sweat during collection. For this reason, the plastic covering the collection gauze should be carefully placed and sealed at its edges. False high values frequently result from failure to exercise deliberate and careful technique.

Interpretation of Results

The finding of a high concentration of sweat chloride is of serious clinical importance, since cystic fibrosis is usually fatal. Even though greatly elevated levels of sweat chloride occur only in cystic fibrosis and the test is very accurate when performed properly, the test should be repeated and the patient's physician conferred with before reporting abnormal results. Normal values range from zero to 30 mEq./L., while patients with cystic fibrosis range from 80 to 150 mEq./L. Marginal values, 50 to 80 mEq./L., sometimes are obtained causing difficulty in interpretation. They should be repeated to insure adequate and accurate collection of sweat. We have obtained marginal values on some patients with Addison's disease, asthma, and severe malnutrition. They have returned to normal following treatment. Parents of children with cystic fibrosis, obligatory carriers, may show significant elevations of sweat chloride, but considerable overlapping with normal individuals is present. There is no method for identification of all heterozygotes at present; thus, the sweat chloride level can not be used in genetic counseling concerning the carrier status.

METHOD

Principle

Sweat glands, in a localized area on the arm or leg, are stimulated by pilocarpine introduced by iontophoresis. The positive electrode is placed on pilocarpine nitrate, the negative electrode at another position on the skin is placed on a suitable current conducting electrolyte. As electrical current is applied, the positively charged pilocarpine radicals move into the skin toward the negative electrode resulting in stimulation of the sweat glands. Special care must be exercised with the negative electrode to avoid electrical burns. After removal of the electrodes, the sweat secreted is collected on weighed gauze. Scrupulous technique is used to prevent contamination by salt or loss of water. The sweat collected averages 0.2 to 0.4 Gm. After suitable elution and dilution of the sweat in the sponge, the sodium content is measured by flame photometry and the chloride content is measured by chloridometer using low concentration standards.

Reagents

1. *Pilocarpine Nitrate Solution*

    Pilocarpine nitrate   1.25 Gm.
    Distilled water, q.s.   250.00 ml.

    Place pilocarpine nitrate in a 250 ml. volumetric flask. Add about half of distilled water to dissolve nitrate. Dilute to volume and store in refrigerator in dark bottle at 46 C. The mixture is usually stable for one month.

2. *Sodium Nitrate*

    Sodium nitrate   1 Gm.
    Distilled water, q.s.   100 ml.

    Dissolve the sodium nitrate in distilled water in a 100 ml. volumetric flask. Dilute to volume.

3. *Stock Sodium Chloride Standard (50 mEq./L.)*

    Sodium chloride   292.5 mg.
    Distilled water, q.s.   1000.0 ml.

    Carefully weigh sodium chloride and place in a 1 L. volumetric flask. Add 500 ml. of distilled water. After the salt goes into solution, dilute to volume.

4. *Working Chloride Standards (1 and 10 mEq./L.)*

    Transfer 1 and 5 ml. of stock standard to 50 and 25 volumetric flasks, respectively. Dilute to volume with distilled water.

Apparatus

Although the power supply for iontophoresis may be constructed from readily available parts, complete instruments may be purchased. Copper is recommended for the electrodes, and they are conveniently made from commercial copper sheet. Copper sheet is relatively pure and a good conductor. Most poorly conductive electrodes and patient "burns" have been associated with steel electrodes. Plastic vials with caps, 1 oz. size, are used for collection and elution containers.

Procedure

Preparation. Exercise care in handling materials used for the collection of sweat since contamination with perspiration from the fingers must be avoided.

Obtain plastic cover squares with sufficient resiliency to withstand child play and abuse. Heavy duty Saran wrap is suitable.

Open package with 2 in. by 2 in. gauze sponges and, using forceps, place one in a clean plastic vial. Replace cap on plastic vial and weigh to the milligram on an analytical balance.

Iontophoresis and Sweat Collection. Plug the power supply into an electrical wall outlet and the leads into the color-coded jacks on the front of the power supply (red = positive terminal; black = negative terminal).

Place the positive electrode (red band around the stem) on a single 3 by 3 in. surgical gauze sponge saturated with 0.5 per cent pilocarpine nitrate solution. Place the negative electrode on a 3 by 3 in. surgical gauze sponge saturated with 1.0 per cent sodium nitrate solution. Place both electrodes in center of their respective sponges to avoid contact with skin.

Select a relatively hair-free area of the inner (flexor) surface of the forearm in older children and adults or the calf area in infants and young children. The latter is a fleshier site which is less easily disturbed by an infant. Place the pilocarpine nitrate positive (red) electrode and sponge on this surface. Place the sodium nitrate negative electrode and sponge on the opposite side. Position both electrodes so that they can be secured by a rubber strap. Secure the electrodes firmly, but without decreasing the circulation in the extremity. Plug the lead connected to the red jack on the power supply into the red-coded pilocarpine electrode on the inner (flexor) surface of the arm. Plug the lead connected to the black jack on the power supply into the negative electrode stem on the opposite side of the arm. Turn the current on by rotating the knob on the power supply in a clockwise direction. Slowly increase the current until the meter reads 1.5 ma. This step should take 1 to 2 minutes, and the patient should feel no pain or shock. However, the patient may notice a mild tingling or prickling. This is harmless and does not require reducing the current.

Turn the current off after 5 to 7 minutes of iontophoresis at 1.5 ma. Remove the electrodes and strap. Allow 5 minutes for the sweat glands to flush out accumulated salt secretions. This is a convenient time to rinse the electrodes with distilled water, as is required after each use. After the 5-minute waiting period, clean the site of the just removed red-coded, positive, pilocarpine-filled electrode with distilled water. Blot dry with a clean 4 in. by 4 in. gauze sponge.

Using forceps, remove the preweighed sponge from the vial and place directly over the skin area of the just removed pilocarpine, red, positive electrode. Place a salt-free plastic cover square over the sponge.

Tape all four sides of the plastic cover square down, using two strips of adhesive tape on each side. Then, cover the exposed center portion of the plastic square with tape as well; this prevents tearing of the plastic cover. The patch must be airtight.

Inform the patient, nurse, or parent that the airtight patch must be worn for one to two hours while the sweat collects on the gauze sponge. During this time the patient is ambulatory and may drink liquids freely unless otherwise contraindicated.

After one to two hours, lift one corner of the patch and quickly remove the sweat-containing sponge with forceps and place it into the plastic vial. Recap the vial. Discard the adhesive tape and plastic cover.

Immediately reweigh to the milligram the recapped vial containing the sweat-soaked gauze.

Calculate the sweat by subtracting the weight of the sponge-vial and cap before collection of sweat from the weight after collection of sweat.

Example:

Weight of vial, cap, sponge and sweat	9.297 Gms.
Weight of vial, cap, and sponge	9.086 Gms.
Therefore: 0.211 Gm. of sweat collected	0.211 Gms.

Chloride Measurement

Pipet 4 ml. of distilled water into vial containing sweat-sponge; recap and mix by inverting. After several minutes, transfer 0.1 ml. of the sponge-eluate to a chloride titrating vial with its measured diluent and indicator. Similarly prepare a distilled water blank and working chloride standards. Titrate each with the chloridometer on low speed. We found that adding the distilled water blank and chloride standards to preweighed gauze containing plastic vials, adding a measured amount of distilled water, and titrating the eluate of each did not enhance accuracy. Thus, this cumbersome practice may be omitted.

Sample calculation:

$$\frac{\text{net titration value of unk.}}{\text{net titration value of std.}} \times \frac{10\,\text{mEq./L.}}{\text{conc. std.}} \times \frac{4.0 + \text{wt. sweat}}{\text{wt. sweat}} = \frac{\text{mEq./L.}}{\text{chloride}}$$

Addendum: In recent months we have obtained experience in measuring the electrical conductivity of sweat and using this measurement as an index of chloride concentration. The conductivity micro-cell is standardized with a series of NaCl solutions (10 to 100 mM/L.); however, the measurement obtained includes other ionic constituents (eg., lactate, potassium, sulfate, calcium) which contribute a lesser portion to the electrical conductivity of the specimen.

In the equipment used,[*] sweat is collected following pilocarpine iotonophoresis. At least 50 mg. of sweat must be obtained in order to fill the special μL microcell, but the small plastic cup supplied for this purpose is satisfactory. When the electrolyte content is very low, a reading is not obtained. We use a sensitive ohmmeter to insure that the microcell is filled with sweat. Though

[*]Cystic Fibrosis Analyzer, manufactured and distributed by Heat Technology Laboratory, Inc., Huntsville, Alabama.

we have observed as much as 16 mEq./L. chloride difference between the conventional sponge-titrimetric and the electroconductivity methods, the latter is suitable for detection of patients with cystic fibrosis.

We have found that by measuring electrical conductivity of sweat in lieu of the sponge-titrimetric method, testing is greatly expedited. Time-consuming careful sponge weighing, sweat elution and chloride titration are circumvented. The electrical conductivity method is now the preferred method for regular use in our laboratory.

REFERENCES

1. Anderson, C. M., and Freeman, M.: "Sweat test" results in normal persons of different ages compared with families with fibrocystic disease of the pancreas. Arch. Dis. Child. 35: 581–587, 1960.

2. Di Sant' Agnese, P. A., Darling, R. C., Perera, G. A., and Shea, E.: Abnormal electrolyte composition of sweat in cystic fibrosis of the pancreas. Clinical significance and relationship of the disease. Pediatrics. 12:549–563, 1953.

3. Gibson, L. E.: Letter-to-editor. Iontophoretic sweat test for cystic fibrosis; technical details. Pediatrics. 39:465, 1967.

4. Gibson, L. E., and Cooke, R. E.: A test for concentration of electrolytes in sweat in cystic fibrosis of the pancreas utilizing pilocarpine by iontophoresis. Pediatrics. 23:545–549, 1959.

5. Shwachman, H., and Antonowicz, I.: The sweat test in cystic fibrosis. Ann. N. Y. Acad. Sci. 93:600–620, 1962.

6. Shwachman, H., and Leabner, H.: Mucoviscidosis. Advances Pediat. 7:249–323, 1955.

CHAPTER XIV

Methemoglobin

Clinical Annotation

HEMOGLOBIN in which iron is in the ferric rather than the ferrous state is called methemoglobin. This compound is not capable of transporting oxygen. Normally there is continuous formation of methemoglobin in the erythrocytes due to various oxidizing substances. There is also an active system for reducing the methemoglobin back to hemoglobin.

Methemoglobinemia is a condition in which a significant proportion of the erythrocyte hemoglobin exists as methemoglobin. Several major types of methemoglobinemia are known, two congenital varieties and an acquired form.

The most common type of congenital methemoglobinemia is due to a defect in the reducing system within the red blood cells dependent upon a normal amount of an enzyme known as methomoglobin reductase. This inborn error of metabolism results in increased amounts of methemoglobin in the red cells. The disease is transmitted via an autosomal recessive gene. With the decrease in oxyhemoglobin the patient usually develops cyanosis and dyspnea. Polycythemia and growth retardation may follow. The increased amount of methemoglobin produced can be readily reduced by the injection of methylene blue.

The second variety of congenital methemoglobinemia is due to a group of rare hemoglobinopathies. The abnormal globulin component in the hemoglobin molecule interferes with the exchange between methemoglobin and hemoglobin. The autosomal dominant variants of this hemoglobin are designated as hemoglobin M (HbM). Several M hemoglobins are known: Boston (HbM_B), Saskatoon (HbM_S), and Milwaukee (HbM_M). The administration of methylene blue or ascorbic acid in these conditions does not convert the methemoglobin pigment to hemoglobin.

Acquired methemoglobinemia is probably more common, especially in pediatric patients. Many chemical agents can induce methemoglobinemia. This is of special importance in infants because fetal (F) hemoglobin is more readily converted to methemoglobin than adult (A) hemoglobin. Therefore, infants with significant amounts of fetal hemoglobin will react to toxic agents at relatively lower doses. The erythrocytes of newborn infants also are relatively deficient in methemoglobin reductase; this adds to the problem. The most frequent drugs involved are acetanilid, antipyrine, and phenacetin. Nitrate and nitrite compounds, occasionally found in water in rural communities, cause formation of methemoglobin. This should be considered in infants presenting with methemoglobinemia, since formula made with such water may be responsible.

Collection Notes

Heparinized or oxalated blood is suitable.

Interpretation of Results

Normal blood usually contains small amounts (1 per cent of total hemoglobin) of methemoglobin. Hospitalized patients may have slightly more methemoglobin (up to 3 per cent of total hemoglobin); this slight increase is unexplained.

Methemoglobin levels of 10 per cent or more are associated with cyanosis, and levels of 30 per cent and above may cause dyspnea, especially if produced acutely. Lethal levels usually are above 75 per cent of the total hemoglobin.

SPECTROPHOTOMETRIC SCREENING FOR METHEMOGLOBINEMIA

Using a recording spectrophotometer, determine the absorption spectrum between 450 and 700 mμ of a hemolysate of red cells in distilled water. Such a curve is shown. Visual inspection of this curve allows one to determine if significant amounts of methemoglobin are present. Since the maximum absorption peaks of all the HbMs occur at significantly different wavelengths, these can be tentatively identified. The usual type of acquired methemoglobinemia is easily recognized on the absorption spectrum. A "shoulder" or peak at 635 mμ is characteristic. Compare the optical density obtained at 635 mμ with that obtained at 675 mμ. If the optical densities at these two wave lengths are essentially the same, no excess methemoglobin is present. If a significant difference in the optical densities is present, excesses of methemoglobin or sulfhemoglobin could be responsible. They can be further differentiated by adding a drop of sodium cyanide to the hemolysate. If the peak is due to methemoglobin, it will be converted to cyamethemoglobin which does not absorb light significantly at 635 mμ, thus the peak will disappear. If the peak persists, sulfhemoglobin may be present.

METHOD

Principle

Methemoglobin has a characteristic optical density peak at 635 mμ. Cyanide abolishes this peak by converting the methemoglobin to cyanmethemoglobin. The difference in optical density at 635 mμ before and after the addition of cyanide is therefore proportional to the amount of methemoglobin.

When the hemoglobin content is known, the amount of methemoglobin can be calculated.

Reagents

1. *Phosphate Buffer, 0.016 M, pH 6.6*

   a. *Sodium Phosphate Solution*

Sodium phosphate, (Na_2HPO_4)	7.1 Gm.
Distilled water, q.s.	500.0 ml.

   Dissolve the sodium phosphate in distilled water and dilute to 500 ml.

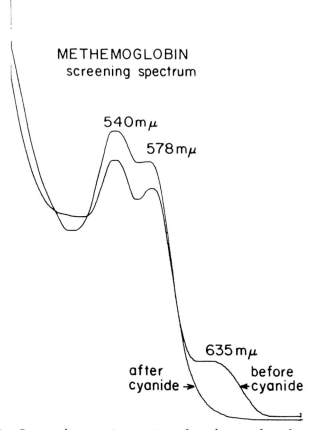

Fig. XIV-1.—Spectrophotometric scanning of erythrocyte hemolysate for methemoglobin.

 b. *Potassium Phosphate Solution*

   Potassium phosphate, (KH_2PO_4) 13.6 Gm.
   Distilled water, q.s.   1000.0 ml.

   Dissolve the potassium phosphate in distilled water and dilute to 1 L.

 c. *Phosphate Solutions Mixture*

   Sodium phosphate solution, (a) 400 ml.
   Potassium phosphate solution, (b) 600 ml.

   Mix solutions together, check pH and adjust to pH 6.6 with remaining solutions as is necessary.

 d. *Phosphate Buffer*

   Phosphate solutions mixture, (c) 166 ml.
   Distilled water, q.s.   1000 ml.

   Dilute phosphate solutions mixture to 1 L. with distilled water and mix thoroughly.

2. *Potassium Ferricyanide*

Potassium ferricyanide	5 Gm.
Distilled water, q.s.	100 Gm.

Dissolve the potassium ferricyanide in distilled water and dilute to 100 ml.

3. *Sodium Cyanide*

Sodium cyanide	5 Gm.
Distilled water, q.s.	50 ml.

Dissolve the sodium cyanide in distilled water and dilute to 50 ml.

4. *Acetic Acid*

Acetic acid, glacial conc.	12 ml.
Distilled water, q.s.	100 ml.

Dilute the acetic acid to 100 ml. with distilled water.

5. *Neutralized Sodium Cyanide*

Acetic acid, 12 per cent	1 ml.
Sodium cyanide, 10 per cent	1 ml.

Add acetic acid to sodium cyanide solution and mix well. This solution is stable for 1 hour.

6. *Methemoglobin Sample*

Fresh heparinized blood	10 ml.
Sodium nitrite, crystals	10 mg.
Ammonium sulfamate	50 mg.

To prepare an intracellular methemoglobin for use as a reagent check, add sodium nitrite to fresh heparinized blood and mix by inversion. Allow to stand 10 minutes. Then add ammonium sulfamate and again mix by inversion. Centrifuge and remove plasma. Wash cells twice with isotonic saline, and then use cells in test determination to check reagents. This specimen will give a greatly elevated methemoglobin content.

Determination of Calibration Factor

1. Determine hemoglobin content of a control sample. (This may be any normal blood sample.)

2. Transfer 0.1 ml. of well-mixed blood into a 12 by 75 mm. cuvet containing 4.0 ml. phosphate buffer (0.016 M) and 0.1 ml. of potassium ferricyanide solution (5 per cent).

3. Mix and allow to stand for 2 minutes.

4. Read optical density ($O.D._1$) at 635 mμ against blank consisting of 4.0 ml. phosphate buffer (0.016 M) and 0.1 ml. potassium ferricyanide (5 per cent).

5. Add 1 drop of neutralized sodium cyanide solution to the sample and the blank.

6. Mix and allow to stand for 2 minutes.

7. Read optical density ($O.D._2$) at 635 mμ of the sample against the blank.

8. Calibration factor $(Fm) = \dfrac{\text{Hemoglobin (Gm. per cent)}}{(\overline{O.D._1 - O.D._2})}$

Substitute this factor into formula for calculating methemoglobin.

Procedure

1. Determine hemoglobin of patient.
2. Transfer 0.1 ml. of well-mixed blood from patient to a test tube containing 3.0 ml. of 0.016 M phosphate buffer.
3. Mix and allow to stand for 2 minutes.
4. Measure optical density $(O.D._a)$ of above solution at 635 mμ against water.
5. Add 1 drop of neutralized sodium cyanide to the entire 3.0 ml. sample. Mix.
6. After 2 minutes measure optical density $(O.D._b)$ against water.

Calculations

Gm per cent methemoglobin $= (O.D._a - O.D._b)\ Fm$

$$\text{percent methemoglobin} = \frac{\text{Gm. percent methemoglobin}}{\text{Gm. percent hemoglobin}} \times 100$$

REFERENCES

1. Evelyn, K. A., and Malloy, H. T.: Microdetermination of oxyhemoglobin, methemoglobin, and sulfhemoglobin in a single sample of blood. J. Biol. Chem. 126:655–662, 1938.
2. Hsia, D. Y.-Y., and Inouye, T.: Methemoglobin, procedure No. 25. In: Inobrn Errors of Metabolism, Part 2 Laboratory Methods. Chicago, Year Book Med. Publ., 1966, p. 44.
3. Miale J. B.: Methemoglobin. In: Laboratory Medicine-Hematology. St. Louis, C. V. Mosby Co., 1958, pp. 262–263.

CHAPTER XV

Cytogenetics

Clinical Annotation

PATIENT EVALUATION and family counseling in genetically determined disorders frequently depends on cytogenetic studies. Such studies were made possible in 1956, when Tjio and Levan correctly described the normal human chromosome complement as 46. It took three more years to dispel the misconception that visible chromosome abnormalities were unlikely to be found. Activity erupted in 1959 when Lejeune and his associates demonstrated constant chromosomal anomalies in mongolism. Since then all the kinds of cytogenetic abnormalities previously observed in experimental genetics have been reported in cultured human cells. Deletions, duplications, inversions, reciprocal translocations, ring chromosomes, single and double trisomies, triploids, and an array of mosaics have been identified. Most of these chromosome abnormalities are associated with aborted embryos or defective children.

Because of the great pressure for more chromosomal analyses of patients in our clinics, we have developed procedures suitable for use in a clinical pathology service laboratory. While research laboratories continue to develop more sophisticated techniques and to discover less obvious cytogenetic abnormalities, the already recognized major anomalies can be discerned and confirmed by the procedures we use or by utilizing a commercial kit.°

Principle

Both the micro and macro methods described in this manual utilize the tissue culture principle for leukocytes in peripheral blood or bone marrow. The cells are incubated in an artificial medium for three days at 37° C., and mitosis occurs when they are stimulated by phytohemagglutinin. Colchicine is used to arrest mitosis in metaphase; then a hypotonic solution serves to spread the chromosomes apart. After fixation and staining, karyotyping is done by microscopic observation with drawing of the metaphase plate or by direct photography with subsequent cutting and arrangement of chromosomes.

Classification of Chromosomes

A karyotype is a systematized array of the chromosomes of a single cell. The Denver grouping and nomenclature is now used by most for arranging the chromosomes of the metaphase plates (karyotyping). A modified schematic karyotype, as proposed by Lennox, is included showing the twenty-two paired autosomes and unpaired sex chromosomes of the male. Although it is idealized, it demonstrates the following group characteristics:

°T C Chromosome Microtest Kit (#5060); T C Chromosome Culture Kit (Macro Method) (#5842). Difco Laboratories, Detroit, Michigan.

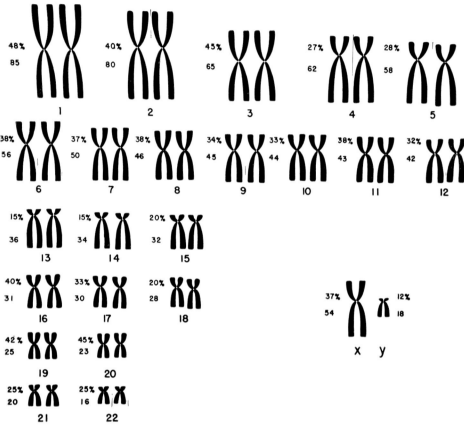

Fig. XV-1.—Chromosome classification.

Group 1 to 3 A	Large chromosomes with approximately median centromeres. The three chromosomes are readily distinguished from each other by size and centromere position.
Group 4 to 5 B	Large chromosomes with submedial centromeres. The two chromosomes are difficult to distinguish, but chromosome 4 is slightly longer.
Group 6 to 12 C	Medium-sized chromosomes with submedian centromeres. The X chromosome resembles the longer chromosomes in this group, especially chromosome 6, from which it is difficult to distinguish. This large group is the one which presents major difficulty in identification of individual chromosomes.
Group 13 to 15 D	Medium-sized chromosomes with nearly terminal centromeres; "acrocentric" chromosomes.
Group 16 to 18 E	Rather short chromosomes with approximately median or submedian centromeres.
Group 19 to 20 F	Short chromosomes with approximately median centromeres.

Table XV-1.—Frequent Autosome Abnormalities

Type of Chromosome Anomaly	Specific Variation	Clinical Characteristics
Numerical alterations:		
Aneuploidy or alteration of number in all cells	Trisomy 21	Down's syndrome
	Trisomy 18	Major physical and mental abnormality: E syndrome
	D Trisomy	Major physical and mental abnormality: D syndrome
	Monosomy	Nonviable
Mosaicism or alteration of number in part of cells	Partial trisomy 21	Variable, perhaps milder than usual Down's syndrome
	Partial monosomy	Occasionally viable
Structural alterations:		
Translocation	15/21 translocation	Translocation carrier or translocation Down's syndrome
	21/21 translocation	Translocation carrier or translocation Down's syndrome
	21/22 translocation	Translocation carrier or translocation Down's syndrome
Deletion	Ring chromosome	Variable
	Deletion of part of short arm of a B chromosome	Cri du chat syndrome
Malignant aneuploidy	Philadelphia chromosome (Ph[1])	Chronic granulocytic leukemia

Group 21 to 22   Very short, acrocentric chromosomes. The Y chromosome is
   G   similar to these chromosomes.

It cannot be overemphasized that it is difficult to select the X chromosome(s) from the similar Group C (6 to 12) chromosomes and to select the Y chromosome from the Group G (21 to 22) chromosomes. Normal females may seem to have sixteen chromosomes in the C group; normal males may seem to have fifteen. In addition, normal males may seem to have an extra chromosome in the G group.

Interpretation of Results

The most common finding in most "service" laboratories is a normal karyotype, the frequency depending on how carefully the patients are screened before studies are undertaken. Because we usually culture leukocytes, we may forget that other tissues do not always give the same picture. Moreover, many lethal conditions are not available for study. The Ph′ chromosome does not appear in fibroblasts, mosaicism for Down's syndrome is more apparent in fibroblasts, and many variations of X-chromosome mosaicism occur in tissues other than leukocytes.

With these reservations, tabulations of the autosomal and X-chromosomal abnormalities readily detectable by leukocyte culture are shown.

Table XV-2.—Frequent Sex Chromosome Abnormalities°

Sex Chromosome Anomaly	Barr Bodies by Buccal Smear	Clinical Characteristics
XO	0	Female, small and asexual
XXX	2	Female, retarded
Xx	1 (small)	Female, abnormal development
xX	1 (large)	Female, abnormal development
XXY	1	Male, small testes, eunochoid
XXXXY	3	Male, retarded and small

°Mosaicism of all the abnormalities listed have been observed.

MICRO-PROCEDURE

Principle

Leukocytes are cultured from 0.1 to 0.2 ml. of whole capillary blood obtained by finger or heel puncture. Two to three drops of blood are allowed to drop into 5 ml. portions of the culture medium. This enriched media consists of Eagle's basal amino acid mixture at double strength in Earle's balanced salt solution. Additives included are glutamine, vitamins, penicillin, streptomycin, phenol red, fetal or newborn bovine agammaglobulin, phytohemagglutinin M, and heparin sodium. pH is adjusted to 7.0 with 7.5 per cent sodium bicarbonate. The cultures are incubated in screw cap vials for three days at 37° C. Colchicine is added for the final three to five hours. After incubation the cells are separated from the medium by centrifugation; then the medium is replaced with dilute sodium citrate solution; the cells are resuspended and allowed to incubate for 20 to 30 minutes. The hypotonic sodium citrate is removed, and the cells are fixed with methanol-acetic acid. The cells are spread on the slide, dried, and stained with Wright's stain. Dehydration and covering of the spread completes the preparation.

Apparatus

Items needed for the procedure are standard. They include a microscope with high resolution lenses, an incubator regulated to 37.5° C., a refrigerator, a centrifuge adjustable to 400 to 800 rpm, and an autoclave. In addition, syringes, needles, microscope slides, cover slips, disposable sterile pipets, screw-capped test tubes (sterile), and new 2 oz. prescription bottles (sterile) are used. All glassware should be scrupulously clean and triple-rinsed with ion-free distilled water.

Reagents

1. Eagle basal medium amino acid mix, (100x).°
2. Eagle basal medium vitamin mix (100x).°
3. Earle's basal salt solution (with phenol red).°
4. L-glutamine.°
5. Fetal bovine serum, agammaglobulin.°

°May be obtained from Microbiological Associates, 4813 Bethesda Ave., Bethesda, Maryland 20014.

6. Phytohemagglutinin, Difco Laboratories, Detroit, Michigan, (dried).
7. Colchicine, Nutritional Biochemicals Corporation, Cleveland, Ohio.
8. Penicillin.
9. Streptomycin.
10. Heparin sodium.
11. Xylene.
12. Wright's stain.
13. Absolute ethanol.
14. Absolute methanol.
15. Permount.
16. Glacial acetic acid.
17. Sodium monophosphate.
18. Potassium diphosphate.
19. Sodium citrate, 1.12 per cent aqueous (w/v).
20. Sodium bicarbonate.

Preparation of Culture Media

(Use sterile precautions throughout procedure.)

1. Autoclave 100 of the 60 by 28 mm. screw cap vials and store sterile.

2. Mix 50 ml. of Earle's basal salt solution (BSS) with 450 ml. of distilled water.

3. In a separate flask, add 10 ml. of Eagle's amino acid mixture to 240 ml. of the BSS prepared in Step 2 for a total volume of 250 ml.

4. In a third flask, add 10 ml. of Eagle's vitamin mixture to 240 ml. of the prepared BSS.

5. Combine Eagle's amino acid and vitamin solutions in a separate 500 ml. volumetric flask.

6. Into another 500 ml. flask, pour about 100 ml. of the combined Eagle's amino acid-vitamin solution. This is the final mixture flask into which all additives are placed.

7. Add 5 ml. of a 200 mM (aqueous) glutamine solution.

8. Add penicillin; required amount is 50,000 units. Add the amount in the smallest volume available. Penicillin should be reconstituted on the day media is made.

9. Add 0.05 Gm. streptomycin. This should be dissolved in BSS prior to putting it into the final mixture flask.

10. Add 75 ml. fetal bovine serum, agammaglobulin to flask.

11. Add 10 ml. of reconstituted phytohemagglutinin.

12. Add heparin sodium; required amount is 10,000 units/500 ml. Add this in the smallest available volume.

13. Fill the flask to the 500 ml. mark with the combined Eagle's amino acid vitamin solution. Adjust pH to 7.0 with 7.5 per cent $NaHCO_3$. Discard the excess, about 90 ml., of Eagle's amino acid-vitamin solution.

14. Pour 5 ml. aliquots of medium into the 100 sterile vials and store frozen ($-20°$ C.).

Culture Procedure

1. Wash finger or heel of patient; dry with ether or air.

2. Obtain 0.1 to 0.2 ml. of whole blood (3 free-flowing drops) by capillary puncture.

3. By direct drops, innoculate the 5 ml. vial of thawed medium with 0.2 ml. of whole blood (3 free-flowing drops).

4. Incubate the culture for three days at 37° C. The cultures are inspected and gently agitated once a day. If the inspection shows the medium has become too acid (color change of indicator from red-orange to orange) loosen screw cap to allow exchange with room air and continue incubation. It takes about two to four hours for the medium color to return to the original red-orange. Mitoses are consistently seen in higher frequency in cultures from some donors when the incubation temperature is elevated to 38 to 39° C.; in rare cases, the same phenomenon is present at temperatures below 37° C. Thus, it may prove worthwhile to incubate different cultures from the same donor at two or more temperatures.

5. On Day 3, colchicine is added to stop cell division in metaphase. Colchicine solution is prepared by adding 10 mg. of colchicine to 1000 ml. of distilled water. Add 0.56 ml. of this solution to the culture.

6. Place the culture in the incubator for three to five hours.

7. Remove the culture from the incubator and transfer the entire mixture by pipet into a 15 ml. siliconized graduated conical tip centrifuge tube.

8. Sediment the cells by centrifugation at 800 rpm for 10 minutes. Centrifuge longer if cells are not spun down after this period as indicated by a cloudy supernatant.

9. Remove the supernatant and replace with 10 ml. of 1.12 per cent sodium citrate which has been warmed to 37° C. Filter through Whatman No. 1 paper before each use to remove bacterial contaminants.

10. Resuspend the cells in sodium citrate. Incubate for 20 to 30 minutes. This salt solution is more gentle in its action and gives better results than the previously used potassium chloride.

11. Centrifuge at 600 rpm for 10 minutes. Spin longer if necessary.

12. Remove the hypotonic sodium citrate and replace with 5 ml. of a freshly prepared 3:1 mixture of absolute methanol and glacial acetic acid. This fixative must be freshly made, as methyl acetate forms rapidly even at refrigerator temperatures. For convenience, we store the methanol-acetic acid mixture at −10° C. in a freezer.

13. Suspend the cells in the fixative *at once* by gentle agitation with a pipet. Failure to do this immediately often results in clumping of cells with poor fixation of the chromosomes.

14. Centrifuge at 800 rpm for 10 minutes or longer if necessary. Resuspend in 3 to 5 ml. of fixative. Now place suspension in refrigerator for a minimum of 15 minutes to insure that fixation be complete. The interval may be extended to several hours or overnight, provided that freshly made fixative is used for the final change.

15. The cells are resuspended and centrifuged at 600 rpm for 10 minutes or longer. An easily dispersed white precipitate should be obtained.

16. Discard the supernatant and add the final fixative—about 0.5 to 1.0 ml. Following the last change of fixative, all traces of color from the hemoglobin should have disappeared.

Slide Preparation

1. Use clean slides.
2. Dip slides in cold distilled water. Air dry.
3. Pipet a few drops of the cell suspension onto the slide. Drain off excess by tilting.
4. Flame the slide.
5. Immerse slide in clean xylene for 15 minutes.
6. Immerse slide in clean methanol for 1 minute.
7. Stain with Wright's stain.

MACRO-PROCEDURE

Principle

The method is essentially the same as for the micro method, except a larger volume (10 ml.) of blood is obtained and a leukocyte-rich portion is used to innoculate the media. Thus, a venipuncture is required to obtain sufficient sample.

Apparatus

Same as for micro procedure.

Reagents

1. Bacto-phytohemagglutinin M- or P (Difco).
2. Sterile water, 5 ml. ampules. Diluent for No. 1.
3. Heparin (1000 units/ml.).
4. Culture medium to TC 199 or NCTC 109.
5. Cochicine (USP) or Colomide (Ciba).
6. Buffered saline solution. Diluent for No. 5.
   a. Sodium chloride (Merck biological to avoid silver contamination).
   b. Sodium biphosphate ($Na_2HPO_4 \cdot 2 H_2O$).
   c. Potassium dihydrogen phosphate ($KH_2 PO_4 \cdot 2 H_2O$).
   d. Calcium chloride.
   e. Phenol red, 0.2 per cent aqueous solution.
7. Sodium citrate 1.12 per cent aqueous solution (w/v).
8. Fixing solution; 1:3 glacial acetic acid in methanol (v/v), freshly mixed.
9. Wright's stain.
10. Absolute alcohol.
11. Xylene.
12. Permount.
13. Penicillin G, aqueous crystalline, 2000 units/ml.
14. Streptomycin sulfate, aqueous, 2 mg./ml .

Preparation of Culture Media and Culture Procedure

1. Stock Buffered Saline:

    a. Dissolve 1.4 Gm. of $CaCl_2$ in 200 ml. of distilled water.

    b. Dissolve 80 Gm. NaCl, 4 Gm. KCl, 0.6 Gm. KH_2PO_4, and 0.6 Gm. $Na_2HPO_4 \cdot 2 H_2O$ in 100 ml. of 0.2 per cent phenol red aqueous solution. Adjust volume to 800 ml. with distilled water.

    c. Combine solutions a and b; then add water to make 1100 ml.

    d. Obtain working buffered saline solution by diluting the stock solution 1:10. Sterilize under 10 lbs. of steam pressure at 115°C. for 10 minutes.

2. Obtain 10 ml. of venous blood in a heparinized syringe and transfer to a sterile screw cap tube. CAUTION: Do not let the blood foam, as the slightest amount of hemolysis interferes with the procedure. The tubes are placed upright in a refrigerator for two to three hours to allow sedimentation of red cells.

3. Place 5 ml. culture medium (TC 199 or NCTC 109) and 0.05 ml. bacto-phytohemagglutinin in a 2 oz. sterile prescription bottle. The addition at this point of 100 units of aqueous crystalline penicillin (0.05 ml.) and 10 mg. of streptomycin sulfate (0.05 ml.) is optional.

  4. Aspirate approximately 2 ml. of leukocyte-rich plasma from the specimen and add to the culture medium. Stopper the prescription bottle and agitate gently.

5. Incubate at 37.5° C. for sixty-eight to seventy-two hours, or incubation may be postponed for as long as three days without losing the specimen if the bottles are placed in a refrigerator.

6. At the end of the first incubation period (seventy hours), add 0.25 ml. of colchicine in saline to the culture. Mix the cultures gently and incubate for three more hours.

7. Pour the culture into a siliconized 15 ml. graduated conical centrifuge tube and centrifuge for 10 minutes at 800 rpm. Then pour off the supernatant.

8. Place 10 ml. of warm (37° C.) 1.12 per cent sodium citrate solution in the original culture bottle and agitate gently to remove any cells that may have adhered to the glass.

9. Add several drops of citrate solution from the culture bottle to the cell button in the centrifuge tube. Suspend the cells by gentle agitation, then add the rest of the citrate solution.

10. Further incubate the cell suspension for 15 to 25 minutes at 37.5° C.

11. Centrifuge the cell suspension at the end of the incubation period for 10 minutes at 800 rpm, then discard the supernatant.

12. Disperse the cell button by adding, dropwise, the freshly prepared cold fixing solution (reagent 8) until approximately 5 ml. has been added.

13. Centrifuge the suspension and discard the supernatant fixative. Add fixative, as in the previous steps, twice more. The cells are now ready for preparation of slides.

Slide Preparation

1. Prepare new slides by cleaning them with 70 per cent alcohol. Add 4 to 5 small drops of the cell culture suspension on the slide and allow them to

CHROMOSOMES

1. METAPHASE

HOMOLOGOUS PAIR

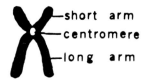
- short arm
- centromere
- long arm

CHROMATID

2. ANAPHASE

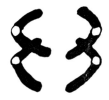

DAUGHTER CHROMOSOMES

POSITION OF CENTROMERE

 median

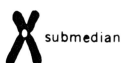 submedian

acrocentric

FINE STRUCTURE

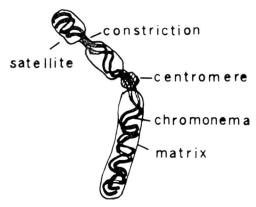
- constriction
- satellite
- centromere
- chromonema
- matrix

Fig. XV-2.—Morphologic characteristics of chromosomes. From Wilson, G. B. Outline of Genetics. Lansing, Michigan State University Press, 1952.

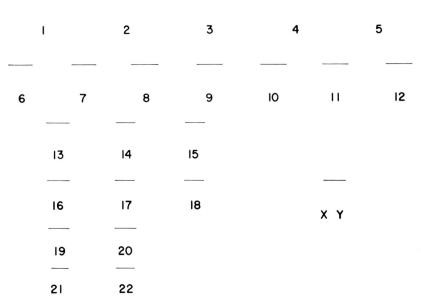

Fig. XV-3.—Outline for preparing human karyotype.

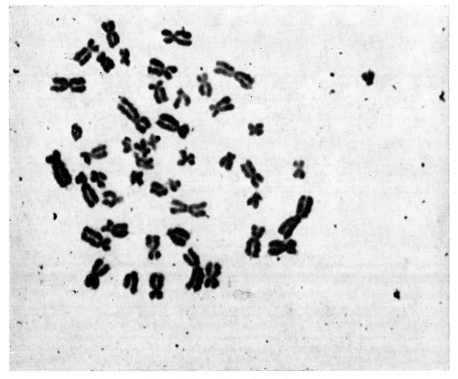

Fig. XV-4.—Metaphase plate.

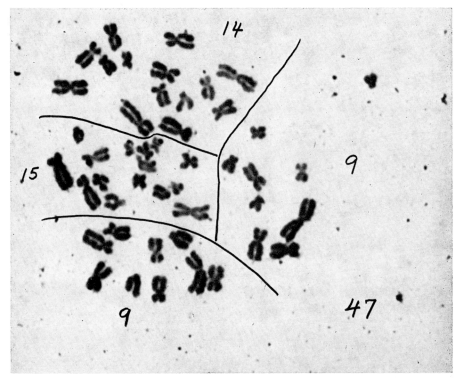

Fig. XV-5.—Chromosomes grouped for easy counting demonstrating abnormal number (47).

spread for about 1 to 2 seconds. Ignite the whole slide with a Bunsen burner or a match. Allow the blaze to extinguish itself. Shake off the few remaining drops of moisture by tapping slide on its side. Allow the slides to dry completely before staining.

2. For staining, Wright's stain is used as for a routine blood smear.

3. Dip the slides in absolute alcohol and then twice in xylene; apply cover slips with permount.

KARYOTYPING

1. Outfit the microscope with the green filter. The monochromatic light improves the contrast of the stained chromosomes.

2. Select a well-spread metaphase without a ruptured cell membrane for counting.

3. Draw several lines to group the chromosomes on a sheet of paper. Start counting.

4. Re-examine each group and select those chromosomes easy to identify which belong to the groups listed below:

    a. Group 13 to 15, or D, medium sized and acrocentric, often referred to as the large acrocentrics; group these first. There are six chromo-

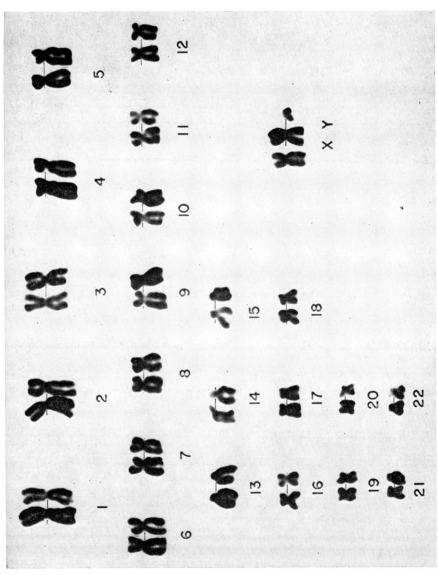

Fig. XV-6.—Karyogram of metaphase plate XV-4 identifying the additional X chromosome.

somes in this group, and they have definite wishbone shapes.

b. Chromosomes of Group 1 to 3, or A, the largest chromosomes. These can be easily identified and numbered.

c. Group 21–22, or G, and the Y chromosome, if present, being the smallest and acrocentric, are easily counted and identified as a group. Four are normally seen in the female, five in the male.

d. The small X-shaped chromosomes are grouped next as 19 to 20, or F.

e. From the remaining complement, the two largest chromosomes with a pincer shape are identified as Group 4 to 5, or B.

f. This leaves Group 16 to 18, or E, and Group 6 to 12, or C, to be classified by size as best as possible.

REFERENCES

1. Denver Study Group (17 members): A proposed standard system of nomenclature of human mitotic chromosomes. Eugenics Quart. 7:96–100, 1960.

2. Denver Study Group (17 members): A proposed standard system of nomenclature of human mitotic chromosomes. J.A.M.A. 174:159–162, 1960.

3. Ferguson-Smith, M. A.: The techniques of human cytogenetics. Amer. J. Obstet. Gynec. 90:(suppl.) 1035–1054, 1964.

4. Ford, C. E., and Hamerton, J. L.: The chromosomes of man. Nature (London). 178: 1020–1023, 1956.

5. Hungerford, D. A.: Leukocytes cultured from small inocula of whole blood and the preparation of metaphase chromosomes by treatment with hypotonic KCl. Stain Techn. 40: 333–338, 1965.

6. Lejeune, J., Gautier, M., and Turpin, R.: Etude des chromosomes somatiques de neuf enfants mongoliens. C. R. Acad. Sci. 248:1721–1722, 1959.

7. Lipfert, A. T.: Technique of human chromosome counts. *In* Gardner, L. I. (Ed.): Molecular Genetics and Human Disease. Springfield, Charles C. Thomas, 1961, pp. 182–185.

8. Lennox, B.: Chromosomes for beginners. Lancet. i:1046–1051, 1961.

9. Moorhead, P. S., Nowell, P. C., Mellman, W. J., Battips, D. M., and Hungerford, D. H.: Chromosome preparations of leukocytes cultured from peripheral blood. Exp. Cell Research. 20:613–616, 1960.

10. Scherz, R. G., and Louro, J. M.: A simple method for making chromosome slides. Amer. J. Clin. Path. 40:222–225, 1963.

11. Tjio, J. H., and Levan, A.: The chromosome number of man. Hereditas (Lond). 42:1–6, 1956.

12. Tjio, J. H., and Whang, J.: Chromosome preparations of bone marrow cells without prior in-vitro culture or in-vivo colchicine administration. Stain Techn. 37:17–20, 1962.

13. Warkany J., Weinstein, E. D., Soukup, S. W., Rubinstein, J. H., and Curless, M. C.: Chromosome analyses in a children's hospital; selection of patients and results of studies. Pediatrics. 33:290–305, 454–465, 1964.

14. Zellweger, H.: Indications for chromosomal analysis in mongolism. J. Iowa Med. Soc. 56:1221–1226, 1966.

Index